Electrotherapy Clinical Procedures Manual

NOTICE

Medicine is an ever-changing science. As new research and clinical experiences broaden our knowledge, changes in treatment and drug therapy are required. The authors and publisher of this work have checked with sources believed to be reliable in their efforts to provide information that is complete and generally in accord with the standards accepted at the time of publication. However, in view of the possibility of human error or changes in medical sciences, neither the authors nor the publisher nor any other party who has been involved in the preparation or publication of this work warrants that the information contained herein is in every respect accurate or complete, and they disclaim all responsibility for any errors or omissions or for the results obtained from use of the information contained in this work. Readers are encouraged to confirm the information contained herein with other sources. For example and in particular, readers are advised to check the product information sheet included in the package of each drug they plan to administer to be certain that the information contained in this work is accurate and that changes have not been made in the recommended dose or in the contraindications for administration. This recommendation is of particular importance in connection with new or infrequently used drugs.

Electrotherapy Clinical Procedures Manual

THERESA NALTY, MS, PT, NCS

Trilogy Consultation & Research
Kent, WA

Assistant Professor
Department of Physical Therapy
University of Texas
Health Science Center at San Antonio

With Contributions By

MOHAMED SABBAHI, PhD, PT, ECS

Professor of Physical Therapy & Neuroscience
Texas Woman's University, Houston

McGraw-Hill

MEDICAL PUBLISHING DIVISION

New York   St. Louis   San Francisco   Auckland   Bogota   Caracas   Lisbon
London   Madrid   Mexico City   Milan   Montreal   New Delhi
San Juan   Singapore   Sydney   Tokyo   Toronto

McGraw-Hill

A Division of *The* **McGraw·Hill** *Companies*

ELECTROTHERAPY CLINICAL PROCEDURES MANUAL

1234567890   DOCDOC   09876543210

ISBN 0-07-134317-2

This book was set in Caledonia by Circle Graphics.
The editors were Stephen Zollo, Lester Sheinis, and Scott Kurtz.
The production supervisor was Catherine Saggese.
The cover designer was Pehrsson Design.
The interior designer was Robert Freese.
The interior illustrations and an illustration on the front cover were by Theresa Nalty.
The index was prepared by Kathrin Unger.

RR Donnelley/Crawfordsville was printer and binder.

This book is printed on acid-free paper.

Library of Congress Cataloguing in Publication Data
Electrotherapy clinical procedures manual / Theresa Nalty ; with a contribution by Mohamed Sabbahi.
      p. cm.
   Includes bibliographical references and index.
   ISBN 0-07-134317-2
      1. Electrotherapeutics—Handbooks, manuals, etc. I. Sabbahi, Mohamed.
   [DNLM: 1. Electric Stimulation Therapy—methods WB 495 N173e 2001]
   RM873.E44 2001
   615.8′45—dc21   00-055030

CONTENTS

Preface   *vii*

1   Introduction   1

2   Electrical Stimulation to Strengthen Muscles   29
or to Prevent Atrophy

3   Electrical Stimulation to Enhance Bone Healing   67

4   Electrical Stimulation to Enhance Circulation   89

5   Electrical Stimulation to Promote Wound Healing   105

6   Nerve Conduction Velocity   131

7   Late Waves   175

8   Electrical Stimulation of Denervated Muscles   209

9   Electrical Stimulation of Abnormal Muscle Tone   215

10   Electrical Stimulation of the Spinal Cord-injured   229
Person

11   Electrical Stimulation of the Stroke Patient   253

12   Pediatric Electrotherapy   273

Index   *301*

Dedication

To JC and His Father. All that I do, I do it for You.

Acknowledgments

The primary motivation for writing this book began while working in a neurological rehabilitation unit. I noticed that many therapists depended on the orthopedic and sports medicine protocols provided by manufacturers of electrical stimulation devices after receiving a prescription for "electrical stimulation." Some therapists became easily convinced that one electrical stimulation device could provide the parameter settings needed to effectively treat all types of patients. With vendor protocols in hand, these therapists felt confident applying electrical stimulation to a patient until they discovered that the parameter settings and subject diagnoses reported in the published article could not be applied to the patient population they were treating. As a clinician I compiled and shared with my colleagues many protocols from the research literature to validate the parameter settings I used to successfully rehabilitate neurologically impaired clients. To this end, I thank my colleagues for opening my eyes to the trap we often fall into when a vendor promotes their product. It is important to remember that we, as practicing medical providers, are responsible for interpreting the research articles and determining the parameters of electrical stimulation best suited for each patient.

I wish to acknowledge Frank Netter, MD, the best medical illustrator of our time, who took the time to smile, squeeze my hand, look into my eyes, and encourage me to follow my dreams.

This book would not have been possible without the guidance and encouragement provided to me by Ron Scott, MSPT, JD, OCS.

A special thanks to my editor Steve Zollo for "taking the heat" when Murphy's Law interfered with meeting deadlines.

To students and clinicians so that they may "Do no harm."

For my children, Christopher and Christina, for sacrificing our shared time in the evenings, on weekends, and on holidays so that this book could be completed.

To my parents and brothers for instilling a sense of love, respect, trust, competition, and camaraderie.

PREFACE

This book provides a valuable resource to the clinician who prescribes or administers electrical stimulation as a therapeutic modality. The concise format used for reporting the electrical parameters is consistent for each chapter so the clinician can rapidly access the information. The majority of the parameter settings are derived from research articles published in peer-reviewed medical journals. Line drawings are provided for an accurate visual reference for electrode placement. It is the *responsibility of the clinician* to determine the optimal protocol for the patient or client based on his/her clinical judgment and area of expertise.

This book was written to aid the busy clinician in determining the best protocol for electrical stimulation for the patient, rather than depending on the convenience of protocols supplied by the manufacturer of the electrical device. The reader of this text will be able to make an informed decision for medical treatment based on recent clinical research on human subjects, rather than relying on studies performed on rats, dogs, pigs, rabbits or *in vitro* laboratory specimens, all of which have differing rates of nervous system recovery, signal transmission, and processing. In addition to the complete medical journal reference, the clinician will have, at his/her fingertips, all of the pertinent research information regarding the sample size, age of subjects, diagnosis, electrical stimulation parameters, number of treatment sessions, and the statistical outcome of the human study.

For many clinicians, the technology and terminology pertaining to the application of electrical stimulation in the clinic has changed since the time of their formal education. With the advent of more sophisticated electrical stimulation units, the clinician now has more control over the parameter settings. This book is intended to bridge the gap between the limited protocols that were once the basis for all patient scenarios and the recent discoveries based on clinical studies with human subjects. The organization and format of this material permits the student and clinician to quickly retrieve the pertinent information needed to accurately set the electrical stimulation parameters for the insurance of optimal patient outcomes utilizing a problem-based approach. Each chapter is independent of the previous chapter and contains an introduction of the material with references for further reading. This knowledge base will ensure consistency in patient care and documentation of electrical stimulation parameters. This handbook is not intended to be the primary teaching tool for the electrical stimulation course in school, but should serve as an adjunct text in the classroom and an essential tool in the clinic.

Topics such as the treatment of pain, sports injuries, or the application of iontophoresis are not included in this handbook because of the multitude of information already in press. Rather, the focus of this book is on the recent developments in electrical stimulation of orthopedic or neurologic conditions. A chapter has been devoted to the review of the literature pertaining to electrical stimulation of the denervated muscle, however; protocols for this procedure have not been provided, due to the author's interpretation of the adverse effect of some protocols on the regeneration of the nerve. The reader is advised to carefully consider the results of research studies where animals or laboratory preparations were used to base the results of effectiveness of electrical stimulation for the human subject due to the differences in the function of the nervous system across species of animals.

Diagnosis of radiculopathy, neuropathy, nerve injury, or other conditions that affect transmission of electrical signals in the nerve falls under the practice act of several professional licenses. While most of this information is available from a variety of textbooks and research articles, the information contained in this handbook is presented in a manner that will enable the clinician to access and apply the testing procedure readily in the clinic.

This handbook is intended to empower the clinician in the use of electrical stimulation for diagnosis and treatment of clients with orthopedic or neurologic impairments. Problem-based organization of the chapters with outcome studies from peer-reviewed scientific studies on human subjects will enhance communication between doctors, therapists, third party payors, researchers, and vendors.

Theresa Nalty
October 2000

Introduction

The use of electricity on a patient requires care in the selection and examination of both the patient and the equipment. It is the responsibility of the clinician to choose the correct form of electricity based on the patient's condition and diagnosis. Electrotherapy has been used for decades to treat a wide range of musculoskeletal and nervous system disorders (Table 1–1). This book is intended to be a clinical handbook to guide the clinician in the selection of the proper current, waveform, amplitude (intensity), and frequency (rate) of electrical stimulation in order to produce the optimal therapeutic outcome for the patient.

In neurophysiologic testing (nerve conduction velocity and late wave responses), *intensity* is used to describe the current flowing from the stimulator and *amplitude* is used to describe the waveform observed on the oscilloscope or screen. In the application of electrical stimulation for treatment purposes, however, the term *amplitude* is preferred when describing the current flowing from the stimulator (Section on Clinical Electrophysiology, 1990). Similarly, the experts in neurophysiologic testing use the term *rate* when describing the current in pulses or cycles per second, whereas the preferred term when describing the same parameter in treatment protocols is *frequency*.

There are many conditions that contraindicate the use of electricity on a patient. Similarly, there are other conditions that were once considered too risky for electrotherapy but that can now be treated successfully if the clinician follows specific precautions and monitors the patient frequently (Table 1–2).

TABLE 1–1
Uses of Electrotherapy

To increase muscle strength
To improve motor control
To stimulate denervated or transplanted muscle
To prevent disuse atrophy
To increase joint range of motion
To reduce edema
To increase circulation
To reduce abnormal muscle tone (spasticity)
To reduce muscle spasm
To increase sensory awareness
To increase speed and precision of movement
To prevent disuse atrophy during immobilization
To facilitate active muscle contraction
To promote wound healing
To improve postural alignment
To provide an orthotic substitution
To assist with walking, bike riding, or other cardiovascular activities
To stimulate bone growth
To relieve pain
To administer drugs across the skin
To reduce tremor and improve hand function

TABLE 1–2
Precautions and Contraindications to the Use of Electrotherapy

Precautions	Contraindications
In hypertensive patients (monitor blood pressure)	Over thoracic area of patients with demand cardiac pacemakers
In patients with arrhythmias due to conduction disturbances or those with congestive heart failure (ECG* first time of electrotherapy)	In regions of phrenic nerve, sacral nerve, or dorsal root stimulators
In third trimester of pregnancy after labor has begun, TENS* may be used to decrease pain	In region of Baclofen pump or other infusion system
Seizure disorder	Over the lumbar, abdomen, or perineal area of pregnant woman
Autonomic dysreflexia	On patients who are unable to provide clear feedback (infants, confused patients, aphasic, head-injured patients)

TABLE 1–2
Continued

Precautions	Contraindications
Sensory loss (such as with a spinal cord injury, multiple sclerosis, etc), frequent skin inspection needed	Over muscles where contraction will adversely affect surgical repair (incision, ligamentous attachment, tendon transfer)
Peripheral neuropathy	In regions of neoplasm
Deep internal fixation (near bone)	
Peripheral vascular disease	In regions with venous or arterial thrombosis or thrombophlebitis
Cardiac patients: monitor for signs of dizziness, shortness of breath, palpitations, and syncope during and after electrotherapy	External fixators, Ilizarov devices, or superficial internal fixation (plates, screws, nails, wires, etc) if forceful muscle contraction will occur
In areas of excessive adipose tissue	Near indwelling arterial lines or near the subcutaneous port used for dialysis
Recent surgery on muscle, tendon, or ligament: surgeon approval for active exercise of area suggests readiness for supervised electrotherapy at low amplitude	Over the eye
Guillain-Barré, multiple sclerosis, postpolio syndrome (do not allow muscle fatigue)	In areas of joint contracture with bony (hard) end feel
Osteoporosis	Over scar tissue
Peripheral nerve injury	Over anterior neck to avoid stimulation of the vagus or phrenic nerve
Allergic reaction to gels, tapes, or electrodes used in electrotherapy	Myasthenia gravis (Ach depletion), Charcot-Marie-Tooth (peripheral neuropathy)
Tissues vulnerable to hemorrhage or hematoma	Over or close to an incision site if muscle contraction would occur
Over thoracic area of thin, small patients	Near operating diathermy devices
Over the head or neck area if history of CVA*	Osteogenesis imperfecta

(*continued*)

TABLE 1–2
Continued

Precautions	Contraindications
On patients with impaired cognition	Active electrode over bruise or bony prominence
If condition that may be exacerbated by increased circulation	Active hemorrhage
On fearful patients, especially if submersion of electrodes part of the treatment	Over irritated or broken skin, unless performing electrotherapy for wound healing
On the immature nervous system (pediatric)	
Fracture in area with less than 6 weeks of healing	

NOTE: There may be other conditions that are contraindicated or require precaution with the use of electrical stimulation.

* ABBREVIATIONS: CVA, cerebrovascular accident; ECG, electrocardiogram; TENS, transcutaneous electrical nerve stimulation.

A thorough examination of the patient is important to verify that the patient is a good candidate for electrotherapy. A careful history should be taken to screen for any contraindications to the use of electricity. A sample examination form may include the following items:

Examination

Patient Name _____   Date of Examination _____
Diagnosis _____   Date of Onset _____
Referring Physician _____
Date Referral Expires _____

History

Past Medical History (Circle all that are true. Write date of onset and comment on line.)

1. Hypertension, autonomic dysreflexia _____
2. Congestive heart failure or conduction disturbance _____

3. Peripheral vascular disease, deep vein thrombosis, pulmonary embolus _____

4. Diabetes: type 1, type 2 _____
5. Guillain-Barré, postpolio, myasthenia gravis, multiple sclerosis

   _____

6. Allergies (list) _____
7. Bone integrity: fracture in area less than 6 weeks, osteoporosis

   _____

8. Neoplasm in area _____
9. Seizure disorder (list medications and describe seizure's
   presentation) _____
10. Brain injury, stroke, central nervous disorder, or disease (list)

   _____

11. Peripheral nerve injury _____

Past Surgical History *(Circle any that apply.)*

12. Pacemaker, phrenic stimulator, sacral stimulator, Baclofen
    pump, dorsal root stimulator _____
13. External fixators (Ilizarov, etc) _____
14. Internal fixation (plates, screws, etc) and location: _____

Social History

15. Alcohol use (list frequency) _____
16. Drug use (name drug and list frequency) _____
17. Educational level _____
18. Occupation _____

Previous Electrical Stimulation

19. Previous use of electrical stimulation
    Type of current and waveform, if known _____
    Date of service _____
    Duration of treatment _____
    Number of total sessions _____
    Response to treatment _____

    _____

20. Patient goals: _____

   _____

Objective Findings of Examination

21. Cognitive status (orientation, affect, ability to follow commands,
    safety, fear) _____
22. Communication _____
23. Skin integrity: abrasions, bruises, scars _____

24. Sensory status (light touch, pain). If deficit, describe and draw area affected _____

25. Neuropathy (document the location) _____

26. Circulatory status (venous thrombosis, thrombophlebitis, Burger's disease, etc) _____

27. Edema (record initial findings using volumetric measurements or circumferential measurements) _____

28. Women: Menses now_____ Pregnant _____

29. Height and weight _____

30. Muscle tone (hypertonic, hypotonic, etc)
Effect of changes in position on muscle tone
Supine _____
Prone _____
Sitting _____
Walking _____
Other purposeful movements _____

31. Motor status (manual muscle test [MMT], coordination) _____
_____

32. Range of motion (ROM) (list abnormal end-feel or contracture-limiting ROM) _____

Equipment Selection and Safety

Inspection

All electrical equipment used on patients should be inspected semi-annually by a biomedical engineer in accordance with Joint Commission on Accreditation of Health Organizations/Commission on Accreditation of Rehabilitation Facilities (JCAHO/CARF) regulations. Equipment used frequently in the clinic should be inspected six times a year (Robinson and Snyder-Mackler, 1995). Any damage to the equipment or exposure to moisture should result in immediate inspection by the engineer before patient contact is allowed. The clinician should examine the cords, plugs, switches, dials, electrodes, wires, and wall outlets prior to each use on a patient. If any of these components are found to be damaged, they should be replaced by qualified personnel immediately. If the device has a large leakage current and the clinician touches both the grounded case of the medical device and the patient at the same time, a serious electric shock to the patient may occur (Mysiw and Jackson, 1997).

The patient treatment area should not contain exposed water pipes, radiators, or other equipment within reach of the patient. The patient treatment area should not be within 3 m (about 10 ft) of microwave or diathermy devices (Robinson and Snyder-Mackler, 1995). Three-prong wall outlets with a ground fault-interrupt (GFI) or equipment with double insulation using Underwriters' Laboratories Standard are required. Do not use two-to-three prong converter plugs or extension cords. Surge protectors in the power lines or at the outlets are also needed. Inspect all equipment prior to bringing the patient into the area.

Electrode Selection

There are many types of electrodes on the market. Carbon rubber electrodes are not disposable and require an even layer of conducting gel for use. The electrode should be secured to the skin in such a way that even pressure is exerted across all points on the electrode. Self-adhesive disposable electrodes should be examined visually before each use for signs of indentations or tears in the conductive surface. If the electrode is not very sticky, a drop of water spread thinly over the surface may renew the sticky texture. If this does not work, discard the electrode. These electrodes should be stored in a sealed bag, which is labeled with the patient's name. Sponge electrodes are used often for large areas, such as the leg or back. The sponges are removed and moistened in water prior to use on the electrode. After use, the electrodes and sponges should be soaked for 20 minutes in a disinfecting solution, such as two-third ounces of Mikro-Quat (ECOLAB Inc, 370 N Washington St, St Paul, MN 55102) in 1 gallon of water (Kalinowski et al, 1996).

The force of muscle contractions induced with surface electrodes is influenced by electrode size and alignment. The size of the stimulating electrode depends on the size and mass of the muscle to be stimulated. A large electrode will distribute the current over a larger surface area, but it may stimulate other nearby muscles. Larger surface electrodes result in a more forceful muscle contraction (Mysiw and Jackson, 1997) and are often used on large muscles of the leg or arm. Smaller electrodes require less amplitude of current because as the electrode size decreases, the current density increases (Myklebust and Kloth, 1992). Current density is the amount of current flow per cubic volume. The current density is highest where the current passes from the electrodes to the skin (Benton and Baker, 1981). If there is adipose tissue, the current density will be decreased en route to the nerve. Charge density, expressed in coulomb per centimeter squared (c/cm²), is the electrical charge per cross-sectional area of the electrode (Section on Clinical Electrophysiology, 1990).

Electrode Placement

Placement of the electrodes parallel to the longitudinal alignment of the muscle fiber length increases the tolerable muscle torque by 64% as compared to alignment of the electrodes in a 90° orientation to the muscle fibers (Lake, 1992). In other words, the current flow should be parallel to the direction of the muscle fibers (Shriber, 1975). Close spacing of the electrodes causes the current to pass superficially across the tissue, whereas increased spacing of the electrodes promotes deep penetration of the current (Benton, 1981). Thus, spacing the electrodes too close together will not only increase the current density to a level of possible tissue injury and pain, but will not stimulate the nerve. The electrodes should be at least as far apart as the diameter of one electrode (Hays, 1993).

The active electrode should not be placed over scar tissue or bony prominences due to higher impedance than normal skin. An electrochemical burn could result at the junction between the normal skin and the area of high impedance (DeVahl, 1992). Electrode placement over adipose tissue may be ineffective and uncomfortable for the patient.

Locating a Trigger Point or Motor Point

Surface electrodes are most often placed over the motor points of muscles if the purpose of electrotherapy is to induce a muscle contraction. Alternatively, trigger points may be used as an electrotherapy focal point for pain management secondary to muscle spasms or connective tissue disorders.

The clinician can become part of the electrical circuit to locate or treat a trigger point or a motor point. The clinician attaches an electrode to his or her left forearm or hand and the other electrode to the patient. The clinician's gel-coated right index finger, touching the patient, completes the electrical circuit, and, thus, acts as the stimulating electrode (Kahn, 1994). The clinician should turn the amplitude up slightly until the patient reports a slight tingling sensation. To identify a trigger point, the clinician lightly moves his or her finger across the patient's reported area of tenderness until a localized region is identified by an increase in sensation in the clinician's right index finger. To locate a motor point, the clinician can move his or her right index finger across the estimated motor point area for the muscle until the exact point is noted where the maximum muscle contraction is obtained. See Figs. 1–1a through 1–1f on pages 10–14 for the motor points.

General Procedures

Once the patient has entered the treatment area, explain the purpose and potential benefits of electrotherapy. Show the patient the equipment to be used, and explain the procedure in order to alleviate fears the patient may have about electrotherapy. Obtain the patient's consent for treatment. Position and drape the patient appropriately. In the area where the electrodes will be placed, cleanse the patient's skin with alcohol or mild soap and water. Skin that is irritated, scratched, or bruised should not have an electrode placed over it. It is important to adhere to the following safety rules: Plug the unit into the socket. Turn the amplitude dial to zero. Turn on the power. Inspect the electrodes, leads, and electrical cords carefully. Connect electrodes to the unit using approved lead wires. Apply electrodes to the patient. Describe the sensations the patient should experience and differentiate these from abnormal or unexpected sensations. Gradually increase the amplitude, being careful to do so only during the on-cycle. Do not adjust more than one parameter at a time. Do not provide moist treatments in conjunction with electrotherapy unless the manufacturer has documentation on the safety for such use. Provide the patient with a call button or emergency stop switch for the duration of the treatment. Instruct the patient not to touch the machine or any other grounded items while the machine is on. Return to check on the patient within the first 5 minutes to adjust the amplitude. When the treatment is completed, turn the amplitude down to zero. Remove the electrodes from the patient, but do not pull the electrodes up using the lead wire. Turn the power off. Disconnect the machine, but do not pull on the cord to unplug it from the socket. Check the patient's skin for irritation or allergic reaction. Document any redness that does not disappear within 15 minutes.

Figures 1–1a to 1–1f   Locations of the Motor Points*

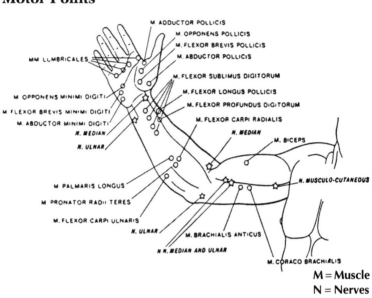

Figure 1–1a

M = Muscle
N = Nerves

* From Prentice WE. *Therapeutic Modalities for Allied Health Professionals.* McGraw-Hill, New York, 1998; pp 506–508.

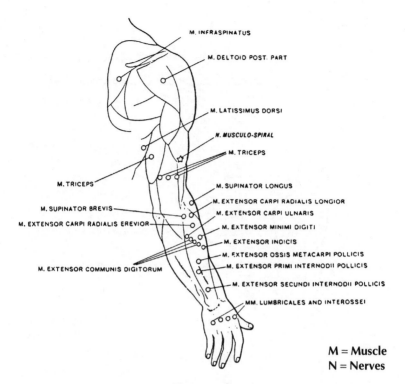

M. INFRASPINATUS

M. DELTOID POST. PART

M. LATISSIMUS DORSI

N. MUSCULO-SPIRAL

M. TRICEPS

M. TRICEPS

M. SUPINATOR BREVIS

M. EXTENSOR CARPI RADIALIS EREVIOR

M. EXTENSOR COMMUNIS DIGITORUM

M. SUPINATOR LONGUS

M. EXTENSOR CARPI RADIALIS LONGIOR

M. EXTENSOR CARPI ULNARIS

M. EXTENSOR MINIMI DIGITI

M. EXTENSOR INDICIS

M. EXTENSOR OSSIS METACARPI POLLICIS

M. EXTENSOR PRIMI INTERNODII POLLICIS

M. EXTENSOR SECUNDI INTERNODII POLLICIS

MM. LUMBRICALES AND INTEROSSEI

M = Muscle
N = Nerves

Figure 1–1b

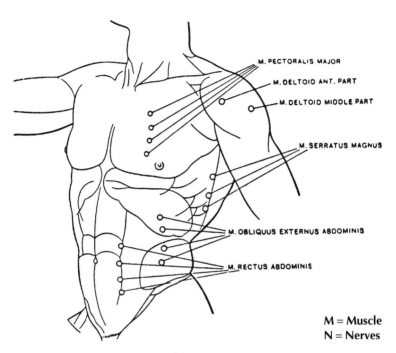

M = Muscle
N = Nerves

Figure 1-1c

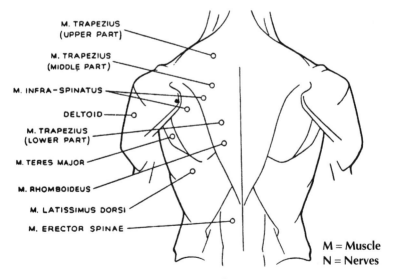

M = Muscle
N = Nerves

Figure 1-1d

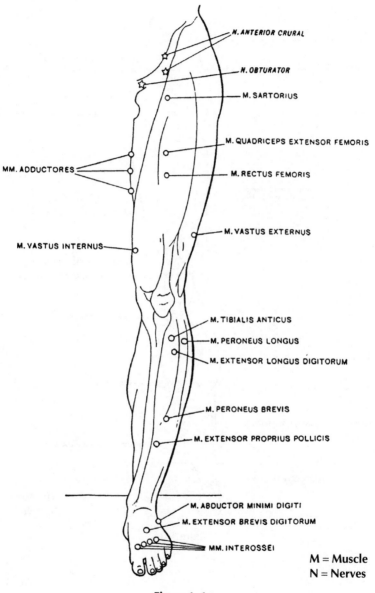

M = Muscle
N = Nerves

Figure 1–1e

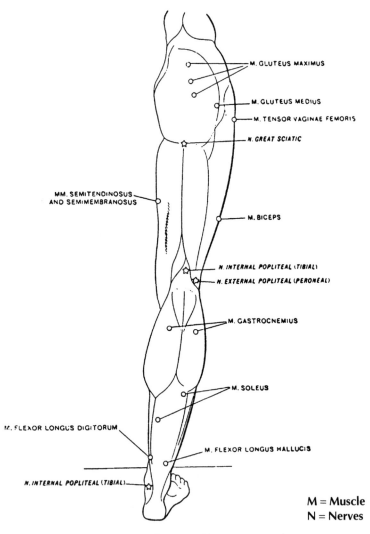

M. GLUTEUS MAXIMUS

M. GLUTEUS MEDIUS

M. TENSOR VAGINAE FEMORIS

N. GREAT SCIATIC

MM. SEMITENDINOSUS AND SEMIMEMBRANOSUS

M. BICEPS

N. INTERNAL POPLITEAL (TIBIAL)

N. EXTERNAL POPLITEAL (PERONEAL)

M. GASTROCNEMIUS

M. SOLEUS

M. FLEXOR LONGUS DIGITORUM

M. FLEXOR LONGUS HALLUCIS

N. INTERNAL POPLITEAL (TIBIAL)

M = Muscle
N = Nerves

Figure 1–1f

If using reusable electrodes, store them in a sealed bag labeled with the patient's name.

Documentation of Electrotherapy

It is important to document all the treatment parameters and effects so that another clinician can reproduce the electrotherapy treatment. Include the device manufacturer, model name and number, the current (biphasic or monophasic), waveform, polarity, number of channels used, and the location of the active electrode(s). The documentation should also include the treatment parameters: amplitude, frequency, pulse duration (previously called pulse width), on/off-time (do not confuse with duty cycle), ramp-up/down-time (do not confuse with rise time/decay time), and duration/frequency of treatment. In addition, the clinician should describe the patient position and details about the electrode, such as the manufacturer's name and the type of electrode. Finally, describe the exact size and anatomic location of each electrode without using the confusing terms "monopolar" and "bipolar" electrode placement (Myklebust, 1992; Nelson and Currier, 1987; Section on Clinical Electrophysiology, 1990).

Polarity

Current flows from the anode (positive electrode) to the cathode (negative electrode). The strength of a muscle contraction produced when the anode is positioned over the motor point is only about 70% of the force produced when the same amplitude of current is applied through the cathode placed over the same motor point (McNeal and Baker, 1988). Thus, a muscle contraction requires less current if the stimulus is applied through the cathode, where depolarization of biologically excitable tissue occurs (Pfleuger's law) (Pfleuger, 1858). The cathode is often referred to as the active or negative electrode and may have a black or white lead wire. Conversely, the anode, usually with a red lead wire, is referred to as the inactive or positive electrode. Depending on the type of circuit, the inactive electrode may be called the dispersive or reference electrode.

The polarity of the electrode is important for certain applications of electrical stimulation. Direct current (monophasic constant current) is used to include a positive potential around a superficial wound to stimulate healing. This is achieved by the use of direct current with varying polarity of the active electrode based on the stages of wound healing. The clinician must pay careful attention to the polarity of the electrodes when applying direct current because even low amplitudes can cause mild acidic reactions under the anode with serious alkaline reactions under the cathode.

In contrast to the acidic potential under the anode, the cathode is of an alkaline nature. In a direct current (monophasic constant current) application, the cathode may be used to soften tissue, dilate tissue, and increase circulation.

Parameters

There are many descriptors for electrotherapy pertaining to the current, the waveform, the number of phases in a waveform, the symmetry of the phases, the balance of the phase charge, the frequency, the pulse duration, the phase duration, the interval, and the amplitude. Each electrotherapy device on the market provides detailed information on each of these areas. The sales representative cannot make a medical decision about which parameter should be changed for each patient diagnosis. The clinician must be able to choose the correct electrotherapy device based on the current and waveform characteristics and must then adjust the parameters according to published data in the medical literature. This clinical guide provides these guidelines and the references where the clinician may find the entire publication. In order to understand the multitude of devices on the market, a brief description of each of the parameters will follow. The clinician should seek textbooks on the matter for a more detailed description of these terms (De Vahl, 1992; Hays, 1993; Kahn, 1994; Mysiw and Jackson, 1997; Nelson and Currier, 1987; Robinson and Snyder-Mackler, 1995; Selkowitz, 1999).

Phase

The phase refers to the direction of current flow for a defined period of time. The monophasic waveform (i.e., monophasic constant current or direct current) has only one phase that deviates in one direction from the baseline and returns to the baseline (Fig. 1–2). Monophasic constant current is the continuous unidirectional flow of charge during which the waveform characteristics do not change over time (DeVahl, 1992; Myklebust and Kloth, 1992; Mysiw and Jackson, 1997). There are

Monophasic Waveform

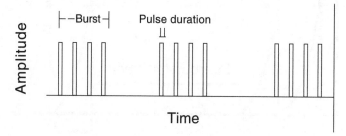

Figure 1–2   Monophasic waveform

voltage fluctuations in response to impedance changes at the interface between the electrode and the patient's skin. If the current is interrupted and monophasic, it is referred to as monophasic pulsed current (Fig. 1–2). The phase duration and the pulse duration in this case are the same. High voltage pulsed current has a characteristic waveform of pulsed monophasic twin-spikes (Fig. 1–3). "Galvanic" is no longer used in conjunction with this form of current (DeVahl, 1992; Myklebust and Kloth, 1992; Section on Clinical Electrophysiology, 1990).

In contrast, the biphasic waveform deviates in one direction from the baseline (one phase) and then deviates in the opposite direction from the baseline (the second phase) before the pulse is complete. An uninterrupted bidirectional flow of charge with reference to the baseline (DeVahl, 1992; Myklebust, 1992) is sometimes called alternating current (AC). When the biphasic current (AC) is not pulsed, the frequency is reported in cycles per second (hertz, Hz); however, in the case of the biphasic pulsed current, the frequency is reported in pulses per second (pps) and includes both phases (Nelson and Currier, 1987). Figure 1–4 illustrates biphasic pulsed current, previously called "interrupted" alternating current (Section on Clinical Electrophysiology, 1990). Note that the pulse duration of a biphasic waveform includes the duration of both phases within the pulse, whereas the pulse duration of a monophasic waveform has only one phase.

A biphasic waveform may be symmetrical or asymmetrical. The symmetrical biphasic waveform has the same amplitude and duration on

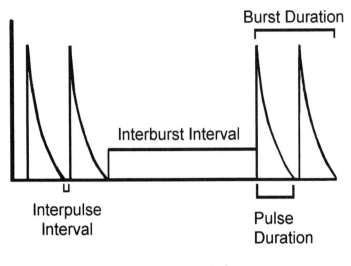

High Voltage Pulsed Current

Figure 1–3 High voltage pulsed current

both sides of the baseline (Fig. 1–4). The symmetrical biphasic square waveform, preferred for stimulation of large muscle groups, has been reported to be more comfortable for the patient than the monophasic waveform at amplitudes high enough to produce a muscle contraction (DeVahl, 1992; Myklebust and Kloth, 1992).

In the asymmetrical biphasic waveform, the amplitude and/or the duration of one phase is unequal with respect to the phase on the other side of the baseline. The asymmetrical biphasic square waveform is clinically effective in the recruitment of smaller muscles (De Vahl, 1992; Myklebust and Kloth, 1992); under the cathode. The asymmetrical biphasic waveforms may be balanced or unbalanced (Fig. 1–5).

In a balanced asymmetrical waveform, the area under the curve of the first phase (above the baseline) is equal to the area under the curve of the second phase (below the baseline). In the unbalanced asymmetrical biphasic waveform, however, the time integral for current in the first phase is *not* equal in magnitude to the time integral in the second phase (Figs. 1–5 and 1–6). Tissue irritants can accumulate under one of

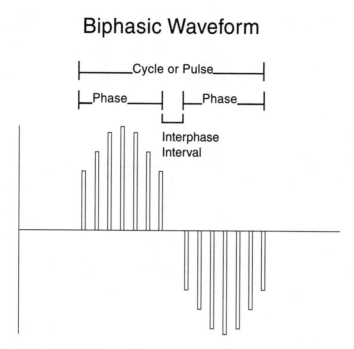

Figure 1–4   Biphasic waveform

the electrodes resulting in burning or itching under the stimulating electrode (De Vahl, 1992; Myklebust and Kloth, 1992). Historically, the term *faradic* was used to describe an unbalanced asymmetrical biphasic waveform (De Vahl, 1992; Myklebust and Kloth, 1992; Section on Clinical Electrophysiology, 1990).

Frequency

The frequency is the number of pulses per second (pps) for pulsed current (monophasic or biphasic). The frequency for uninterrupted biphasic current (i.e., alternating current) is expressed in cycles per second using the unit of hertz (Hz). Manufacturers and clinicians performing electrophysiologic testing often use the term *rate* for this same variable. The preferred term for application of electrotherapy is *frequency*.

When the frequency of electrical stimulation is 1–4 pps, the patient typically reports a "pins and needles" sensation. Electrical stimulation

Unbalanced Asymmetrical Biphasic Current

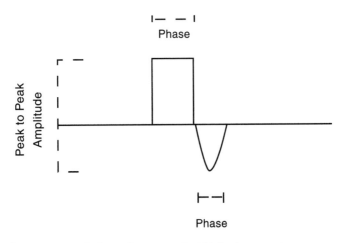

Figure 1–5 Unbalanced asymmetrical biphasic current

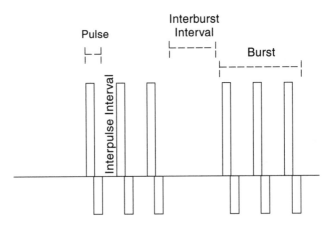

Unbalanced Biphasic Waveform

Figure 1–6 Unbalanced biphasic waveform

applied to the nerve at 5 pps results in a short duration muscle contraction called a muscle twitch and is perceived by the patient as a "tapping" sensation. As the stimulation frequency is increased to 10–20 pps, a vibration-like quality of muscle contraction occurs where the muscle never totally relaxes between contractions. At 25–30 pps, fused tetany occurs. The contractile force produced by a muscle fiber at tetany is four times that of a single muscle twitch. Above 50–70 pps there is no significant increase in muscle tension.

A train is a continuous sequence of pulses (of monophasic pulsed current or biphasic pulsed current) or cycles (of uninterrupted biphasic current) (see Fig. 1–7). This continuous train of pulses or cycles is categorized under the mode of current. Other descriptions for mode of current include interrupted, reciprocate, burst, or beat. A burst is a defined series of pulses or cycles with milliseconds of no current flow separating each burst (see Figs. 1–2 and 1–6). The millisecond period between bursts of pulses or cycles is called the interburst interval. Medium frequency burst AC includes a description for the carrier frequency of the

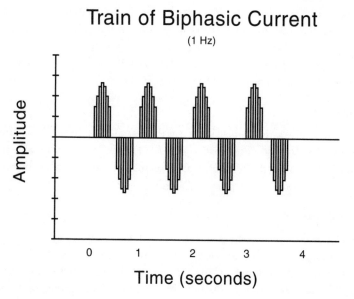

Figure 1–7   Train

biphasic current (usually between 2200 and 2500 Hz), as well as a burst frequency, such as 50 bursts per second.

Duration

Phase duration is the time elapsed from the beginning to the end of one phase of a pulse (Fig. 1–4). Phase was previously defined as the direction of current flow for a defined period of time. A pulse is an isolated electrical event separated by a finite time from the next event (Section on Clinical Electrophysiology, 1990). Thus, a monophasic waveform with only one phase has a phase duration that is equal to the pulse duration. A biphasic waveform has two phases, often of different durations. In the case of a biphasic pulsed current, both phase durations (above as well as below the baseline) are summed to determine the pulse duration.

It has been reported in the literature that a phase duration of 0.3 ms is more comfortable than a 0.05 or 1.0 ms duration (Bowman and Baker, 1985; Gracanin and Trnkoczy, 1975). A possible explanation for this phenomenon is that the wider phase duration of 1.0 ms recruits both motor and pain axons (DeVahl, 1992; Myklebust and Kloth, 1992), whereas the smaller phase duration requires a painfully high amplitude.

Burst durations usually refer to medium frequency burst AC (previously called Russian stimulation) or high voltage pulsed current (see Fig. 1–3). Beat durations usually refer to medium frequency beat AC (sometimes called interferential current).

Interval

The interpulse interval (also known as the intrapulse interval) is the time between pulses (see Figs. 1–3 and 1–6). The interburst interval is the time between bursts (see Fig. 1–3). The interphase interval is the time between two successive phases of a pulse (see Fig. 1–4).

Amplitude

In electrotherapy, "amplitude" is preferred when describing the magnitude of current with reference to the baseline (Robinson and Snyder-Mackler, 1995; Section on Clinical Electrophysiology, 1990). "Intensity" is often used, however, by clinicians performing electrophysiologic testing when referring to the amount of current flowing from the stimulator.

Peak amplitude is the maximum amplitude for each phase. Peak-to-peak amplitude is the summation of the amplitude for both phases above and below the baseline of an alternating current (see Fig. 1–5). Low amplitude devices with a current less than 1 mA are available for the treatment of localized painful areas or trigger points due to muscle spasms or connective tissue disorders. Manufacturers use a multitude of names for this device, including microcurrent electrical stimulation (MES), micro-amperage stimulation (MS), microcurrent nerve stimulation (MNS), microcurrent electrical nerve stimulation (MENS), and, in some cases, low intensity direct current (LIDC) and low intensity stimulation (LIS).

As the amplitude is increased, there is a linear relationship in the number of motor units recruited (Lake, 1992). The large diameter Aα fibers are the first to be recruited as the sensory receptors in the muscle spindle and Golgi tendon organ are stimulated. Once the Aα fibers are stimulated, the Aβ fibers can be recruited by either increasing the pulse duration of the electrical stimulation or increasing the amplitude of stimulation. Aβ fiber stimulation results in a motor response. Once the motor threshold is reached, the clinician should increase the amplitude of electrotherapy very slowly and cautiously to avoid causing pain to the patient. The clinician should also be aware that the painful response, due to recruitment of the Aδ nerves, may also be produced by a very small increase in the pulse duration.

The patient's nervous system will accommodate to the electrical stimulation after about 5 minutes, requiring the clinician to increase slightly the amplitude of electrotherapy in order to maintain the desired level of muscle contraction. In the case of a denervated muscle, the myoneural junction is not intact, requiring the clinician to use direct current if the outcome of electrotherapy is a muscle contraction. In contrast to the response of normal muscle to electrotherapy, as described in the previous paragraph, the denervated muscle requires a higher amplitude, longer pulse duration, or both, to achieve a motor response. The sensory fibers may be intact in a denervated muscle, however, making this high amplitude electrical stimulation extremely painful for the patient.

On/off-times

The time during which a train of monophasic pulses or biphasic cycles, or a series of beats or bursts, are delivered is called the on-time (Fig. 1–8).

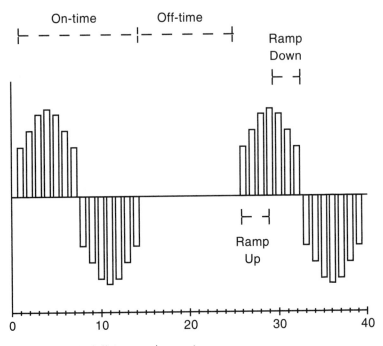

Figure 1–8 On/off-times and ramp times

The time between trains or series of bursts is called the off-time. On/off-times are often reported in the literature as a ratio. For example, 5 seconds on and 15 seconds off is reported in the simplest form as the ratio 1:3. This ratio is often used as a starting point for strengthening the quadriceps muscles of healthy subjects or orthopedic patients (DeVahl, 1992; Myklebust and Kloth, 1992). As strength or endurance improves, the off-time is decreased in order to increase the number of muscle contractions per minute. Alternatively, increasing the off-time is recommended if the patient's muscle easily fatigues. For instance, a 1:5 ratio of 5 seconds on and 25 seconds off has been reported to be the starting point for hemiparetic patients or for use on smaller muscles (DeVahl, 1992; Myklebust and Kloth, 1992; Packman-Braun, 1988).

Duty cycle

The duty cycle is the ratio of on-time multiplied by 100 divided by the sum of on-time plus off-time (DeVahl, 1992; Section on Clinical Electrophysiology, 1990). The duty cycle, which is reported as a percentage, has also been calculated as the pulse train duration multiplied by 100 with the product divided by the total cycle time (DeVahl, 1992). The lack of consistent reporting of the on-time and off-time in terms of the ramp time makes calculation of the duty cycle confusing. It is even more difficult to determine the exact parameters when trying to decipher research articles that only report the duty cycle. For these reasons, the duty cycle is no longer the preferred form of documentation, although it is still reported for descriptions of medium frequency burst AC (formerly known as Russian stimulation).

Ramp-up Time and Ramp-down Time

Most electrotherapy devices offer an adjustable period of time that the stimulus takes to reach peak amplitude (ramp up) and to return from peak amplitude to the baseline (ramp down). The ramp-up time is used to allow the patient to become accustomed to the stimulation as it progresses from sensory to motor thresholds. The ramp-down time allows a gradual release of the muscle contraction (Fig. 1–8). These features more closely simulate a physiologic voluntary muscle contraction. Once a protocol has been established for a patient, increasing the amplitude will cause a steeper ramp-up slope to reach the higher amplitude within the preset ramp-up time. This may cause discomfort for the patient. It is recommended to increase the ramp-up time when increasing the amplitude (Selkowitz, 1999).

On-time and Off-time

Researchers consider any amount of current flow inducing a subsensory, perceivable, or motor response to be the on-time and, thus, would include the ramp-up as well as the ramp-down times. Thus, off-time is the amount of time when no current is flowing (Fig. 1–8). Documentation of the parameters should include a specific on-time of current flow and an off-time (baseline amplitude).

The Relationship of Ramp Time to On/Off-time

Many manufacturers will include both ramp times in the on-time, while other manufacturers will report the on-time as separate from either the ramp-up time or the ramp-down time (Respond Select, EMPI 599 Cardigan Road, St Paul, MN 55126). While it is expected that the ramp-up time and ramp-down time will be reported, it is up to the clinician to contact the manufacturer of the electrical stimulator to verify if the on-time for the device includes the ramp-up time, the ramp-down time, neither, or both. Authors, when describing treatment parameters for electrotherapy, often assume that the on-time is separate from the ramp times (Selkowitz, 1999). Other authors have described the ramp-up time as a part of the on-time, yet describe the ramp down as part of the off-time (DeVahl, 1992). Manufacturers often refer to the on-time as the contraction time, which, depending on the protocol, may not even cause a muscle contraction.

Due to the confusion in reporting this parameter, it is not possible to determine if ramp times or rates significantly influence force output, fatigue, or the strength gain of the electrically stimulated muscle.

Rise Time and Decay Time

While ramp time refers to a gradual change in amplitude over a series of pulses or phases, rise and decay (the latter once called fall or decline) times are used to describe single pulse characteristics (Robinson and Snyder-Mackler, 1995; Selkowitz, 1999). The rise and decay times are often reported for the high voltage pulse current, which consists of a monophasic twin peak pulsed current (see Fig. 1–3). The rise time is the time for the leading edge of the pulse to increase from the baseline to peak amplitude. Similarly, the decay time is described as the time for the trailing edge of the pulse to return to the baseline from the peak amplitude (Section on Clinical Electrophysiology, 1990). Note that both rise and decay times are included in the on-time. When reviewing published articles or manufacturer's specifications, the clinician should be aware that the ramp-up time may be erroneously reported as rise time, just as the ramp-down time is often incorrectly recorded as decay time.

Metric Conversions

Metric conversions, which are necessary for understanding the electro-therapy parameters, can be derived with an understanding of the fol-• lowing relationships:

Amplitude:
100 mA = 0.1A
and 1 mA = 1000 µA
just as 10 mA = 0.01 A = 10,000 µA

Duration:
4 ms = 4000 µs
0.3 ms = 300 µs
0.05 ms = 50 µs

References

Benton LA, Baker LL: *Functional Electrical Stimulation: A Practical Clinical Guide*, 2d ed. Downey, CA, Rancho Los Amigos Rehabilitation Engineering Center, 1981.

Bowman BR, Baker LL: Effects of waveform parameters on comfort during transcutaneous neuromuscular electrical stimulation. *Ann Biomed Eng* 13:59, 1985.

DeVahl J: Neuromuscular electrical stimulation (NMES) in rehabilitation, in MR Gersh, *Electrotherapy in Rehabilitation*, Philadelphia, FA Davis, 1992; pp 218–268.

Gracanin F, Trnkoczy A: Optimal stimulus parameters for minimum pain in the chronic stimulation of innervated muscle. *Arch Phys Med Rehabil* 56:243–249, 1975.

Hayes KW: *Manual for Physical Agents*, 4th ed. Norwalk, CT, Appleton & Lange, 1993; p 88.

Kahn J: *Principles and Practice of Electrotherapy*, 3d ed. New York: Churchill Livingstone, 1994; p 81.

Kalinowski DP, Brogan MS, Sleeper MD: A practical technique for disinfecting electrical stimulation apparatuses used in wound treatment. *Phys Ther* 76(12):1340–1347, 1996.

Lake DA: Neuromuscular electrical stimulation: An overview and its application in the treatment of sports injuries. *Sports Med* 13:320–336, 1992.

McNeal DR, Baker LL: Effects of joint angle, electrodes and waveform on electrical stimulation of the quadriceps and hamstrings. *Ann Biomed Eng* 16:299, 1988.

Myklebust BM, Kloth L: Electrodiagnostic and electrotherapeutic instrumentation: Characteristics of recording and stimulation systems and the principles of safety, in MR Gersh, *Electrotherapy in Rehabilitation*, Philadelphia, FA Davis, 1992; pp 55–64.

Mysiw JW, Jackson RD: Electrical stimulation, in *Physical Medicine & Rehabilitation*, RL Braddom (ed.). Philadelphia, WB Saunders, 1997; pp 469–470.

Nelson RM, Currier DP: *Clinical Electrotherapy*. Norwalk, CT, Appleton & Lange, 1987.

Packman-Braun R: Relationship between functional electrical stimulation duty cycle and fatigue in wrist extensor muscles of patients with hemiparesis. *Phys Ther* 68:51–56, 1988.

Pfleuger EW: Ueber die tetanisierende Wirkung des Constanten Stromes und das Allgemeingesetz der Reizung. *Virchow's Arch* 3:13, 1858.

Robinson AJ, Snyder-Mackler L: *Clinical Electrophysiology: Electrotherapy and Electrophysiologic Testing*, 2d ed. Philadelphia, Williams & Wilkins, 1995.

Section on Clinical Electrophysiology: *Electrotherapeutic Terminology in Physical Therapy*. Alexandria, VA, American Physical Therapy Association, 1990.

Selkowitz DM: Electrical currents, in MH Cameron, *Physical Agents in Rehabilitation From Research to Practice*, Philadelphia, WB Saunders, 1999; pp 345–427.

Shriber WJ: *Manual of Electrotherapy*. Philadelphia, Lea & Febiger, 1975.

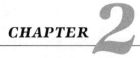

Electrical Stimulation to Strengthen Muscles or to Prevent Atrophy

Electrical stimulation to increase strength in normal innervated muscle is useful in postoperative cases involving immobilization or contraindication to dynamic exercise. Electrical stimulation has been shown to be an effective adjunct to voluntary exercise when pain, swelling, fatigue, or the lack of motor control prevent a strong muscle contraction.

In general, muscle-strengthening protocols use medium frequency alternating currents and a rest period that is five times the stimulation period. The use of medium frequency burst alternating current for muscle strengthening was first proposed in 1977 by a Russian scientist for use on elite athletes (Kots, 1977). This technique, once referred to as Russian stimulation or the Russian technique, uses a carrier frequency of 2200–2500 Hz to deliver bursts of 50–75 per second. Generally, the pulse duration (including both phases of the alternating cycle) is between 50 and 250 μs, but it has been reported to be as high as 1 ms (1000 μs).

The on/off-times may be reported as a duty cycle, which in medium frequency burst alternating current is the ratio of the burst duration (i.e., on-time) to the burst duration plus the interburst interval (i.e., on-time plus off-time). Many clinicians, however, erroneously report the on/off-cycle as a simple ratio and then refer to it as the duty cycle. To add more confusion to the issue, some clinicians include the ramp times in the on-time, other clinicians report the ramp up in the on-time and the ramp down in the off-time, while still other clinicians leave the ramp times out of the calculation altogether. For this reason, the use of the term duty cycle is not recommended. Rather, the actual on- and off-times should be reported. In addition, the ramp times should be clearly documented. See Chap. 1 for further explanation of this calculation.

Fatigue of the electrically stimulated muscle occurs when the on-time is prolonged (18 seconds or more) or if the on:off ratio is 1:1. This ratio is useful for building muscle endurance, but for strengthening without inducing fatigue of the muscle, the off-time should be four to six times that of the on-time (Hosking et al, 1978; Packman-Braun, 1988).

When electrical stimulation is combined with voluntary contraction of the normal muscle, the torque developed is less than that obtained from voluntary isometric contraction alone (Currier, 1991). A comparison of the strength gain following either isometric exercise, electrical stimulation with isometric exercise, and electrical stimulation alone found no significant difference between the three methods when used on the normal quadriceps femoris (Currier and Mann, 1983; Kramer and Semple, 1983; Kubiak et al, 1987; Selkowitz, 1989). The same findings were noted in healthy, nonsurgical subjects in that the knee extensor strength increased in groups that performed isometric exercise at an equivalent amount as those who performed isometric exercise in conjunction with electrical stimulation (Currier et al, 1979). Likewise, there has been no significant difference noted between the quadriceps strength gain with isometric exercise when compared with the gain from electrical stimulation alone (McMiken et al, 1983). McMiken and associates concluded that the therapeutic value of electrically stimulated muscle contractions should be used for patients who are noncompliant, poorly motivated, or who have poor tolerance for near maximal isometric muscle contractions. Similarly, there was no significant difference in the maximum voluntary isometric torque between postoperative knee patients who had performed isometric exercises in conjunction with electrical stimulation of the quadriceps versus a postoperative group who only performed isometric exercise (Grove-Lainey et al, 1983; Lieber et al, 1996; Sisk, 1987).

The current amplitude for muscle strengthening should represent a percentage of the mean values for the pretest maximum voluntary isometric contractions (abbreviated as %MVIC). A more accurate description of the %MVIC would include the duration of the contraction as the "torque/time index." The torque/time index should be used to compare performance for each repetition of an individual (Selkowitz, 1985). Elite athletes, who have not recently been injured or undergone surgery, may be able to tolerate electrical stimulation amplitudes up to 165%MVIC (Selkowitz, 1985); however, studies on postoperative anterior cruciate ligament reconstruction patients have never reported such values. Initially, electrical stimulation of an injured or postoperative muscle should be about 10%MVIC (Selkowitz, 1999). The %MVIC increases over time within each electrical stimulation session, as well as from week to week, thus the amplitude should be gradually increased within each session as well as from day to day (Laughman et al, 1983; Selkowitz, 1989). A large increase in amplitude from one repetition to another may cause discomfort and result in cocontraction of the antagonistic muscle, adversely affecting the torque of the stimulated muscle. Selkowitz (1989) determined that in order for the electrical stimulation groups to produce greater strength gains than the voluntary isometric contraction groups, muscle contractions with greater forces than voluntary movements must be produced. The torque produced during an electrically stimulated contraction is not consistently related to the amplitude of the current, but it is influenced by the patient's tolerance to the electrical stimulation secondary to postoperative status, pain, or motor control capabilities; muscle fatigue at the end of a training session; and the individual's strength limit, as well as the availability of the appropriate electrical stimulation unit (Currier and Mann, 1983; Selkowitz 1989).

The position of the muscle, especially if it crosses two joints, may be crucial for the maximum benefit from electrical stimulation. In addition, greater strength gains have been noted when the position for testing was the same as that used for training with electrical stimulation. For the quadriceps femoris, many authors are reporting significant improvements in isometric strength when a training position of 60° hip flexion (from supine) and 60° knee flexion is used.

Another technique to strengthen muscle using medium frequency electrical current is based on the concept of interference of two currents with different frequencies. This technique, called interferential current or interference current, uses two circuits: one with a fixed carrier frequency of 4000 Hz (4 kHz) and the other with a frequency that can be varied between 4001 and 4100 Hz. The resultant beat frequency to the tissue ranges between 1 and 100 Hz. At intersection frequencies up to 10 Hz, motor nerves are depolarized for mild muscle contractions, which are useful for relaxation and muscle reeducation. As stronger contractions are desired, the intersection frequency may be increased. Because of the narrow phase duration, high amplitudes are needed to elicit muscle contractions, but they may not be effective in producing enough torque for strengthening (Snyder-Mackler et al, 1989). At intersection beat frequencies of 90–100 Hz, the autonomic nervous system is inhibited, which will affect sympathetic tone and will allow comfortable muscle stimulation in the presence of nerve irritation or neuritis. This higher intersection frequency, which is more comfortable due to less skin impedance from the decreased pulse charge, is also useful in treating edema and deep muscle spasms, which are cases where repetitive stimulation is needed (Santiesteban, 1990). Interference current is not unique in the use of high frequency currents to penetrate deeper tissues. Any electric stimulator with the capability of providing a high frequency of alternating current with a pulse duration of less than 100 μs will stimulate deep tissues (Kloth, 1992). This short pulse duration will require a relatively high stimulation amplitude in order to cause a muscle contraction using interference current (Kloth, 1987).

PROCEDURE 2–1

Strengthening of the Normal Quadriceps Femoris

Parameters	Settings
Current type/waveform	Pulsed sine wave
Current amplitude	70 mA (400 V peak-to-peak)
Ramp up	5 seconds
Ramp down	0
Carrier frequency	2500 Hz
Burst modulation (frequency)	50 bursts per second
Burst on-time	10 ms
Burst off-time	10 ms
Total stimulation on-time (including ramp)	15 seconds (10 seconds of muscle contraction)
Rest between stimulation times	50 seconds
Treatment duration	10 repetitions once a day, 5 days/week × 5 weeks
Electrode configuration	13 cm gelled electrodes:
	Proximal: inferior to inguinal ligament, over upper rectus femoris and vastus lateralis
	Distal: distal margin of vastus medialis 5–7 cm superior and medial to the superior pole of the patella

5–7 cm

Strengthening of the normal quadriceps

(*continued*)

PROCEDURE 2–1

Continued

Parameters	Settings
Unit	ElectroStim 180 MicroMed Instruments 4994 Place de la Savane Montreal, Quebec Canada H4P1R6 ElectroStim USA Ltd 1851 Black Rd Joliet, IL 60435

OTHER: Sitting with hip at 60° from supine and knee at 60° flexion.

OUTCOME: Three groups were enrolled in the study: a control group (n = 19), an isometric exercise only group (n = 19), and an electrical stimulation group (n = 20). There was no significant difference between the group performing isometric exercise only and the group receiving electrical stimulation. The isometric exercise group performed 10 second contractions with 50 second rests × 10 repetitions daily, 5 days/week for 5 weeks, and demonstrated an 18% increase in torque.

SOURCE: Laughman RK, Youdas JW, Garrett TR, Chao EYS: Strength changes in the normal quadriceps femoris muscle as a result of electrical stimulation. *Phys Ther* 63:494–499, 1983.

PROCEDURE 2–2

Electrical Stimulation of the Immobilized Leg Following Anterior Cruciate Ligament (ACL) Reconstruction

Parameters	Settings
Current type/waveform	Not reported
Pulse duration	Not reported
Current amplitude	Tetanizing contraction < 100 V
Frequency	200 Hz
On-time	5–6 seconds
Off-time	5 seconds
Treatment duration	1 hour/day, 5 days/week × 4 weeks
Electrode placement	*Proximal:* above femoral nerve in groin area
	Distal: cast window at distal quadriceps

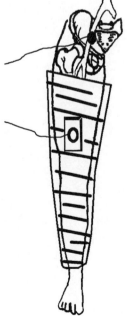

Electrical stimulation of the immobilized leg following anterior cruciate ligament (ACL) reconstruction

(*continued*)

PROCEDURE 2–2

Continued

OUTCOME: Eight subjects randomly assigned to two groups who received muscle biopsies at 5 cm from the vastus lateralis about 15 cm above the patella preoperatively, at 1 week postoperation, and at 5 weeks postoperation. After surgery, all eight subjects were casted from the ankle to the groin with 10° knee flexion. All subjects in both groups performed isometric exercise. Four subjects had cast windows cut over the distal quadriceps for placement of the distal electrode. The group receiving electrical stimulation had less atrophy and better muscle function than the control group. There was a significant difference in the biopsied muscle in that the electrically stimulated muscle had increased levels of succinate dehydrogenase (SDH), whereas the control group did not show any difference in the SDH level. Prevention or the fall in SDH correlates with less muscle atrophy.

SOURCE: Eriksson E, Häggmark T: Comparison of isometric muscle training and electrical stimulation supplementing isometric muscle training in the recovery after major knee ligament surgery. Am J Sports Med 7:169–171, 1979.

PROCEDURE 2–3

Electrical Stimulation Following Anterior Cruciate Ligament (ACL) Surgery

Parameters	Settings
Current amplitude	Maximum tolerated, increased by patient with each cocontraction
Carrier frequency	2500 Hz
Burst modulation	50 bursts per second
On-time	15 seconds
Off-time	50 seconds
Treatment duration	Fifteen cocontractions a day, 5 days/week × 3 weeks
Electrode configuration	Four gelled 4.5 × 10 cm carbon rubber electrodes on the quadriceps:
	(1) proximally over vastus lateralis
	(2) distally over vastus medialis
	(3) over medial hamstring and
	(4) over short head of the biceps femoris

Strengthening following anterior cruciate ligament (ACL) surgery

(*continued*)

PROCEDURE 2–3

Continued

Parameters	Settings
Unit	VeraStim 380 Electro-Med Health Industries, Inc 6240 NE 4th Ct Miami, FL 33138

OTHER: Postoperative orthotic removed during electrical stimulation, which typically began the second or third week postoperatively.

OUTCOME: Twenty subjects, 19–44 years of age, were randomly assigned to two groups. One group received electrical stimulation, and the other group performed the same exercises at maximum knee flexion. The group of 10 patients receiving electrical stimulation had higher percentages of flexion and extension isometric torque at 65° of flexion than those patients performing voluntary exercise only at 4–6 weeks after surgery.

SOURCE: Delitto A, Rose SJ, McKowen JM, et al: Electrical stimulation versus voluntary exercise in strengthening thigh musculature after anterior cruciate ligament surgery. *Phys Ther* 68:660–663, 1988.

PROCEDURE 2–4

Electrical Stimulation of the Quadriceps During Postoperative Immobilization

Parameters	Settings
Current type/waveform	Monophasic pulsed current
Pulse duration	350 µs
Current amplitude	On average: 52 mA
Ramp up	4 seconds
Ramp down	2 seconds
Frequency	50 pps
On-time	10 seconds
Off-time	50 seconds
Treatment duration	On average: 6 hours/day for 36 days over 6 weeks
Electrode configuration	Self-adhering electrodes were moistened and placed proximally over the midline of the quadriceps 15 cm distal to the anterior superior iliac spine (ASIS) and placed distally through cast window on the motor point of the vastus medialis
	Electrodes: Tenzcare (3M, 3M Center, Building 304-1-0, St Paul, MN 55144-1000)

Strengthening of the quadriceps during postoperative immobilization, 45° knee flexion

(*continued*)

PROCEDURE 2–4

Continued

Parameters	Settings
Unit	Respond II EMPI 599 Cardigan Rd St. Paul, MN 55126 (This unit was formerly sold by Medtronic.)

OTHER: Electrical stimulation was initiated 1–3 days postoperatively over the quadriceps with the leg casted at 45° knee flexion.

OUTCOME: Fifteen patients were enrolled in the study and divided into two groups, with eight receiving electrical stimulation through a window in the cast. After 6 weeks, there was a significant difference in the isometric torque changes between the two groups ($P = 0.05$). Those patients in the control group demonstrated a preoperative torque of 168 ft-lb, but dropped 80% in strength to 34 ft-lb of isometric torque at 6 weeks postoperation. The group receiving electrical stimulation dropped from 135 ft-lb to 54 ft-lb, a 60% loss in isometric torque. Strength testing was performed with the patients wearing derotational braces. While there was a measurable change in strength, there was no significant difference for either group in thigh girth when comparing preoperative values to those at 6 weeks.

SOURCE: Morrissey MC, Brewster CE, Shields CL, Brown M: The effects of electrical stimulation on the quadriceps during postoperative knee immobilization. *Am J Sports Med* 13:40–45, 1985.

PROCEDURE 2–5

Low Frequency Electrical Stimulation After Knee Ligament Surgery

Parameters	Settings
Current type/waveform	Biphasic pulsed current, asymmetrical, rectangular waveform
Pulse duration	300 μs
Current amplitude	65–100 mA increased gradually within tolerance
Ramp up	2 seconds
Frequency	30 Hz
On-time	6 seconds
Off-time	10 seconds
Treatment duration	Four 10 minute sessions with 10 minute breaks, three times a week
Electrode configuration	*Proximal:* 5 cm distal to the inguinal ligament
	Distal: window cut in cast for carbon rubber electrode (4 × 10 cm) over the vastus lateralis 10 cm proximal to the upper border of the patella; electrodes were covered with a 0.5 kg weight

Low frequency electrical stimulation after knee ligament surgery

Unit	Respond II EMPI 599 Cardigan Rd St Paul, MN 55126 (This unit was formerly supplied by Medtronic.)

(*continued*)

PROCEDURE 2–5

Continued

OTHER: Postoperative cast for 6 weeks at 20–30° flexion. All patients performed isometric quadriceps contractions in 20–30° knee flexion for 10 minutes every hour, eight times a day. Electrical stimulation was initiated on the second postoperative day. Patients were told to contract quadriceps in conjunction with electrical stimulation.

OUTCOME: Twenty-three patients, 21–45 years of age, were randomly assigned to one of two groups: an electrical stimulation group and a control group. Six weeks postoperatively, the isometric quadriceps strength at 30° flexion had decreased from the preoperative value by 58% for the control group, but by only 39% for the group receiving electrical stimulation ($P < 0.01$)

SOURCE: Wigerstad-Lossing I, Grimby G, Jonsson T, et al: Effects of electrical muscle stimulation combined with voluntary contractions after knee ligament surgery. *Med Sci Sports Ex* 20(1):93–98, 1988.

PROCEDURE 2–6

Electrical Stimulation of the Quadriceps and Hamstrings After Anterior Cruciate Ligament (ACL) Reconstruction

Parameters	Settings
Current type/waveform	Alternating current, triangular waveform
Pulse duration	400 µs
Current amplitude	Maximum tolerated (increased gradually throughout 15 contractions)
Ramp up	3 seconds
Ramp down	None
Carrier frequency	2500 Hz
Burst modulation	75 bursts per second
On-time	15 seconds (includes a 3 second ramp)
Off-time	50 seconds
Treatment duration	Fifteen contractions per session, 3 days/week
Electrode configuration	Four electrodes on same circuit: vastus medialis, vastus lateralis, short head of biceps femoris, and medial hamstrings

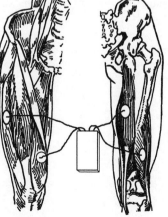

Strengthening of the quadriceps and hamstrings after anterior cruciate ligament (ACL) reconstruction

(*continued*)

PROCEDURE 2–6
Continued

Parameters	Settings
Unit	VeraStim 380 Electro-Med Health Industries 11601 Biscayne Blvd Suite 200A North Miami, FL 33181-3151

OTHER: Electrical stimulation for cocontraction of the quadriceps and hamstrings was initiated at 3–6 weeks postoperatively in one group. Patients in both groups removed the postoperative orthotic and exercised volitionally twice a day, 7 days a week, positioned in 60–90° knee flexion with a 15 second cocontraction of the hamstrings and quadriceps followed by a 50 second rest period. Other standard treatments for both groups included passive range of motion (PROM) exercises at 10° per second times 30 repetitions, isokinetic hamstring exercise at increasing speed (at second week postoperative), and isokinetic cycling for 10 minutes (at fifth week postoperative).

OUTCOME: Ten patients were enrolled in the study and were randomly assigned to two groups. One performed the volitional exercises and received the standard treatment, and the other group received the additional modality of electrical stimulation while positioned in 60° knee flexion. The average isokinetic torque and peak torques for the quadriceps femoris were significantly greater in the group receiving electrical stimulation than the volitional exercise group at 90° per second ($P < 0.05$) and at 210° per second ($P < 0.01$)

SOURCE: Snyder-Mackler L, Ladin Z, Schepsis A, Young JC: Electrical stimulation of the thigh muscles after reconstruction of the anterior cruciate ligament: Effects of electrically elicited contraction of the quadriceps femoris and hamstring muscles on gait and on strength of the thigh muscles. *JBJS* 73(A):1025–1036, 1991.

PROCEDURE 2–7

Electrical Stimulation and Electromagnetic Stimulation After Arthroscopic Anterior Cruciate Ligament (ACL) Reconstruction

Parameters	Settings
Current type/waveform	Alternating current, sine wave
Current amplitude	50%MVIC (based on greatest torque of three preoperative trials)
	On average reached a maximum of 82.6 ± 16.2 mA (range 30–96 mA)
Carrier frequency	2500 Hz
Burst modulation	50 bursts per second, 10 ms on/ 10 ms off
Ramp up	5 seconds
On-time	15 seconds (including ramp up)
Off-time	50 seconds
Treatment duration	Ten contractions per session with instructions to cocontract hamstrings and quadriceps simultaneously with the electrical stimulation. Electrical stimulation initiated within 24 hours of surgery with one session for 3 successive days. Thereafter, the electrical stimulation was administered with the regular physical therapy, three times a week for 5 weeks (for a total of 18 sessions over 6 weeks)
Patient position	For electrical stimulation, the patient sat with the hip at 90° flexion and the knee fully extended
Electrode configuration	Two pairs of carbon rubber electrodes (8 × 12.5 cm) were connected to the same parallel circuit. Wet sponges were used as the conducting medium. One electrode pair was placed on the

(*continued*)

PROCEDURE 2–7

Continued

Parameters	Settings
	femoral nerve in the femoral triangle and over the vastus medialis muscle. The second pair was placed on the belly of the biceps femoris distally and over the medial hamstring proximally.

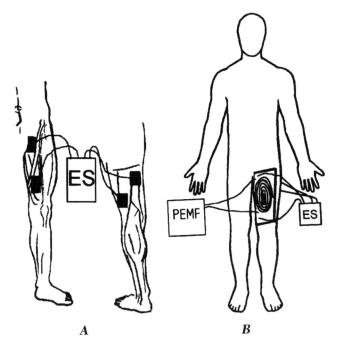

A   B

Electromagnetic and electrical stimulation of the thigh muscles within 24 hours of anterior cruciate ligament (ACL) reconstruction

Electrical Stimulation	Electrostim 180-2i Stimulator
	Electrostim USA Ltd
	1851 Black Rd
	Joliet, IL 60435

PROCEDURE 2–8

Pulsed Electromagnetic Field

Parameters	Settings
Peak amplitude	1.5 Tesla (15,000 gauss) to produce quadricep torque at > 50%MVIC (when combined with electrical stimulation)
Frequency	60 cosine pulses per second
Coil configuration	26 cm coil superimposed over the electrical stimulation electrode pairs
On-time	10 seconds (15 second durations caused intense coil heating) in conjunction with 15 seconds of electrical stimulation for muscle contraction
Treatment duration	5.3 weeks
Electromagnetic stimulation	Cadwell model MES-10 (modified) Cadwell Laboratories, Inc 909 N Kellogg St Kennewick, WA 99336

OTHER: Postoperatively placed in orthotic at 5° flexion for 5–6 weeks. Other standard treatments included ROM exercises, isometric quadriceps and hamstring exercises, straight leg raise exercise, and ambulation within the first 6 weeks postoperatively.

OUTCOME: Seventeen patients (15–39 years of age) were enrolled in the study. Three patients received no electrical stimulation, seven received electrical stimulation only, and seven received electrical stimulation with pulsed electromagnetic field. There was no significant difference in the thigh girth measurements between the group who received electrical stimulation only and the group who received electrical stimulation with pulsed electromagnetic field. The control group, however, experienced a significant loss in thigh girth when compared with either the electrical stimulation group or the electrical stimulation with pulsed electromagnetic field group ($P < 0.01$). Using the visual analogue scale, the patients receiving electrical stimulation with pulsed electromagnetic field reported significantly less pain ($P < 0.01$) than when the electrical stimulation alone was applied (3.4 ± 1.6 cm versus 7.3 ± 1.1 cm, respectively).

SOURCE: Currier DP, Ray JM, Nyland J, et al: Effects of electrical and electromagnetic stimulation after anterior cruciate ligament reconstruction. JOSPT 17(4):177–184, 1993.

PROCEDURE 2–9

Electrical Stimulation of the Patient After Open Meniscectomy

Parameters	Settings
Current type/waveform	Monophasic pulsed current, square wave
Pulse duration	100 μs
Current amplitude	Gradually increased to 100 mA
Ramp up	3 seconds
Frequency	35 pps
On-time	5 seconds
Off-time	2.5 minutes
Treatment duration	16 hours/day × 2 weeks
Electrode configuration	Unique conductive foam 1.26 cm wide with a stainless steel foil and cloth backing. Three electrodes (single channel) were placed circumferentially around the thigh at 8 cm distal to the gluteal fold, 5 cm above the patella, and posteriorly around the widest point of the calf without touching the superficial surface of the tibia. The proximal electrode was positively charged and the middle and distal electrodes were negatively charged. The voltage divider between the middle and distal electrodes allowed only 30% of the current to flow to the calf, whereas; the thigh received approximately 70% of the current.

Circumferential foam electrodes used to stimulate muscles under a knee immobilizer within 24 hours of open meniscectomy

OTHER: Electrical stimulation under the knee immobilizer was initiated the day after surgery.

PROCEDURE 2–9

Continued

OUTCOME: Twenty patients who were treated by open meniscectomy by the same two surgeons were divided into two groups. Both groups performed several hundred quadriceps isometric contractions per day. Strength, ROM, and muscle leg volumes were measured before and at 4 weeks postoperatively (2 weeks after cessation of electrical stimulation). At 4 weeks postoperatively, the average ROM in the control group decreased by 32°, while the average ROM in the stimulated group increased by 40° ($P < 0.05$). Both groups experienced a loss of torque at 4 weeks postoperatively in comparison to the preoperative values, but the control group experienced significantly greater losses in power for the quadriceps, hamstrings, plantar flexors, and dorsiflexors (each muscle $P < 0.05$).

SOURCE: Gould N, Donnermeyer D, Gammon GG, et al: Transcutaneous muscle stimulation to retard disuse atrophy after open meniscectomy. *Clin Orthop Rel Res* 178:190–197, 1983.

PROCEDURE 2-10

Electrical Stimulation of the Postsurgical Immobilized Limb

Parameters	Settings
Current type/waveform	Alternating current
Current amplitude	To tetany
Carrier frequency	2500 Hz
On-time	15 seconds
Treatment duration	Ten repetitions for a total of 150 seconds of stimulation for 6 weeks
Electrode placement	Through cast to the quadriceps

OUTCOME: Three postoperative patients had their affected knees immobilized. After 10 days of immobilization, electrical stimulation was begun. Biopsies of the vastus lateralis muscle revealed that the electrically stimulated group had elevated levels of ATPase, whereas the immobilized control group had ATPase levels that decreased.

SOURCE: Standish WD, Valiant GA, Bonen A, et al: The effects of immobilization and of electrical stimulation on muscle glycogen and myofibrillar ATPase. *Can J Appl Sports Sci* 7:267, 1982.

PROCEDURE 2-11

Electrical Stimulation for Patients With Chondromalacia or Subluxing or Dislocating Patellae

Parameters	Settings
Current type/waveform	Biphasic pulsed current, symmetrical waveform
Current amplitude	As high as tolerated to cause palpable contraction of the vastus medialis and medial translation and counter-tilt of the patella
Ramp up	2 seconds
Ramp down*	1 second
Frequency	30–35 Hz
On-time	10 seconds
Off-time*	30 seconds with progression to 10 seconds, as tolerated over 3 weeks
Treatment duration*	Progress from 15 minutes daily to three sessions a day; increase duration of each session in 10–15 minute increments as tolerated over 2–3 weeks
Electrode configuration	3.0 cm carbon rubber (negative) electrode was placed on vastus medialis about 8 cm proximal to superior aspect of the patella, and anode (4 × 5 cm) was placed just proximal to tibiofemoral line medial to the patella

Electrical stimulation to the vastus medialis in patients with chronically dislocating patellae

* SOURCE: Bay Area Physical Therapy, Oakland, CA.

(continued)

PROCEDURE 2–11
Continued

Parameters	Settings
Unit	Respond
	EMPI
	599 Cardigan Rd
	St. Paul, MN 55126

OTHER: Patient should perform isometric quadricep exercises or terminal extension exercises, with or without ankle weights, during electrical stimulation.

OUTCOME: Case report of a patient with chronic subluxation and dislocation of the patella. Electrical stimulation was applied with the knee in full extension. During electrical stimulation with maximal voluntary isometric contraction of the quadriceps, the patella did not sublux; however, the patella continued to sublux during functional activities when electrical stimulation was not in use. There was no significant change in the lateral displacement forces of the patella as measured with a Chatillon push-pull gauge after 2, 4, or 6 weeks of electrical stimulation of the vastus medialis.

SOURCE: Bohannon RW: Effect of electrical stimulation to the vastus medialis muscle in a patient with chronically dislocating patellae. *Phys Ther* 63:1445–1447, 1983.

PROCEDURE 2–12

Electrical Stimulation to Prevent Extensor Lag Following Total Knee Arthroplasty

Parameters	Settings
Current amplitude	80% of that needed to invoke a visible muscle contraction of the contralateral limb
Ramp up	3 seconds
Frequency	35 Hz
On-time	15 seconds
Off-time	10 seconds
Treatment duration	1 hour, twice a day
Electrode configuration	*Proximal:* over the femoral nerve
	Distal: over the vastus medialis obliquus
Patient position	From 40° knee flexion to full extension with electrical stimulation while in continuous passive motion (CPM) machine

Electrical stimulation to prevent extensor lag in total knee arthroplasty patients

(continued)

PROCEDURE **2–12**

Continued

Parameters	*Settings*
Unit	Mentor Bio Sales, Inc 116 Walnut Ave Cranford, NJ 07016

OTHER: All patients received standard physical therapy, including CPM, to the affected limb, ambulation, ROM and strengthening exercises, and activities of daily living training.

OUTCOME: Forty patients were randomly assigned to either a control group or an electrical stimulation group after receiving a total knee replacement. After electrical stimulation during CPM, the extensor lag was 5.7° compared with an extensor lag of 8.3° for the control group ($P < 0.01$); whereas preoperatively there was no significant difference. In addition, discharge criteria were reached significantly faster in the group receiving electrical stimulation than in the control group ($P < 0.05$).

SOURCE: Gotlin RS, Hershkowitz S, Juris PM, et al: Electrical stimulation effect on extensor lag and length of hospital stay after total knee arthroplasty. *Arch Phys Med Rehabil* 75(9):957–959, 1994.

PROCEDURE 2–13

Electrical Stimulation to Prevent Muscle Atrophy Following Total Knee Arthroplasty

Parameters	Settings
Current type/waveform	Biphasic pulsed current, square wave
Pulse duration	250 µs
Current amplitude	As tolerated for visible contraction
Frequency	30 Hz
On-time	10 seconds in conjunction with CPM cycle
Treatment duration	1.5 hours/day × 7 days
Electrode configuration	Motor points

OUTCOME: Sixteen patients, 61–79 years of age, requiring unilateral total knee arthroplasty for severe osteoarthritis were enrolled in the study. They were randomly assigned to one of two groups: the control group receiving CPM or those receiving CPM with electrical stimulation. The CPM was progressed from 40° within the first 48 hours postoperatively by 10° daily. The addition of electrical stimulation for 7 days prevented marked fiber atrophy as evidenced by nearly identical muscle biopsies pre- and postsurgery. There was a significant difference in the rate of atrophy between the group receiving electrical stimulation and those who received CPM alone.

SOURCE: Martin TP, Gundersen LA, Blevins FT, Coutts RD: The influence of functional electrical stimulation on the properties of vastus lateralis fibres following total knee arthroplasty. Scand J Rehabil Med 23:207–210, 1991.

PROCEDURE 2–14

Electrical Stimulation of the Quadriceps Muscle for Patients Unable to Perform Maximum Voluntary Isometric Contractions (MVIC)

Parameters	Settings
Current type/waveform	Biphasic pulsed current
Pulse duration	0.1 ms
Current amplitude	Gradually increased, but not to exceed 80%MVIC or 10 V
Frequency	75 Hz
On-time	10 seconds
Off-time	50 seconds
Treatment duration	Ten contractions per session, once a day, × 9 days
Electrode configuration	*Proximal:* 120 × 40 mm plate electrode over folded moistened pad was strapped over the quadriceps at the femoral triangle at the motor point for the rectus femoris.
	Distal: 130 × 60 mm plate electrode over folded moistened pad was strapped over the motor point of the vastus medialis

Electrical stimulation of the quadriceps for patients unable to perform a strong voluntary isometric contraction

Patient position	30° knee flexion

PROCEDURE 2–14

Continued

OTHER: Prior to electrical stimulation, the area was washed and then soaked for 5 minutes with a hot towel to reduce skin resistance.

OUTCOME: Fifteen patients, 19–27 years of age, were randomly assigned to either an electrical stimulation group or an isometric exercise group. The isometric exercise group performed 10 second contractions with 50 second rests with the same treatment duration as the group receiving electrical stimulation. Those receiving only electrical stimulation demonstrated a 22% increase in strength as compared with a 25% increase in strength for those performing isometric exercise.

SOURCE: McMiken DF, Todd-Smith M, Thompson C: Strengthening of human quadriceps muscles by cutaneous electrical stimulation. *Scand J Rehabil Med* 15:25–28, 1983.

PROCEDURE 2–15

Prevention or Retardation
of Muscle Atrophy

Parameters	Settings
Current type/waveform	Medium frequency burst AC (Russian stimulation)
Pulse/cycle duration	As close as possible to duration needed for chronaxie of the motor nerve
Current amplitude	25%MVIC
Carrier frequency	2500 Hz
Burst modulation	20–85 bursts per second
On-time	6–15 seconds
Off-time	At least 1 minute, preferably 2 minutes
Treatment duration	15–20 minutes with at least 10 contractions up to three sets of 10 contractions, twice a day
Electrode configuration	*If small muscles:* one channel with two electrodes
	If large muscles: two channels with four electrodes

OTHER: Muscle should be given some resistance (gravity, weighted limb, or fixed motion isometric)

SOURCE: Hooker DN: Electrical stimulating currents. In: Prentice WE, *Therapeutic Modalities for Allied Health Professionals.* McGraw-Hill, New York, 1998, p 99.

PROCEDURE 2–16

Electrical Stimulation of the Forearm Post-Colle's Fracture: A Case Report

Parameters	Settings
Current type/waveform	Biphasic pulsed current, asymmetrical waveform
Pulse duration	300 μs
Current amplitude	To fair/fair plus muscle contraction
Ramp up	4 seconds
Ramp down	2 seconds
Frequency	30 pps
On-time	12 seconds
Off-time	12 seconds
Treatment duration	Increase as tolerated to 15 minutes, 3 times a day × 5 weeks
Electrode	4.6 × 4.6 cm carbon-silicon
Electrode configuration	*Channel one:* proximal third of forearm over the extensor muscle belly with the second electrode on distal forearm 5 cm proximal to the wrist crease
	Channel two: proximal upper third of the forearm over the flexor muscle belly with the second electrode over the flexor tendons about 8 cm proximal to the wrist crease

Electrical stimulation after cast removal following a Colle's fracture

(*continued*)

PROCEDURE 2-16

Continued

Parameters	Settings
Company	Medtronic Nortech Division San Diego CA 92121

OTHER: Electrical stimulation was not initiated until after cast removal. Other modalities included hotpack, ultrasound, use of the Baltimore Therapeutic Exercise (BTE) work simulator, mobilization, ROM exercises, hand-strengthening exercises with putty, active and active-assisted hand exercises, and ice.

OUTCOME: After 5 weeks of electrical stimulation and the above treatment, the patient demonstrated 90% of the normal range of motion for the wrist and fingers.

SOURCE: Stralka SW: Application of therapeutic electrical currents in the management of the orthopedic patient, in *Electrotherapy in Rehabilitation,* MR Gersh (ed.). FA Davis, Philadelphia, 1992, pp 355–361.

PROCEDURE 2–17

Electrical Stimulation to Increase Abdominal Strength

Parameters	Settings
Current type/waveform	Biphasic pulsed current, symmetrical
Pulse duration	200 μs
Frequency	50 Hz
On-time	5 seconds for week 1 7.5 seconds for week 2 10 seconds for week 3 12.5 seconds for week 4
Off-time	5 seconds for week 1 7.5 seconds for week 2 10 seconds for week 3 12.5 seconds for week 4
Treatment duration	3 times a week × 4 weeks
Electrode configuration	Rubber electrodes shaped to contour the entire abdominal area

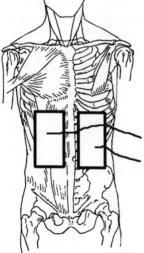

Electrical stimulation of the
abdominal muscles

(*continued*)

PROCEDURE 2–17
Continued

Parameters	Settings
Unit	Intellect VMS prototype
	Chattanooga Corp
	Chattanooga, TN

OUTCOME: Thirty-two patients, 20–40 years of age, were randomly assigned to one of four groups: a volitional exercise group, an electrical stimulation group, a volitional exercise in conjunction with electrical stimulation, or a control group. Abdominal muscle endurance was measured at 45° trunk flexion in units of time. Average abdominal strength was measured with a force transducer during three maximal voluntary isometric contractions. The electrical stimulation group was significantly stronger at the end of the second week than the control or volitional exercise groups. The group receiving electrical stimulation in conjunction with volitional exercise demonstrated a greater percent mean increase of %MVIC over pretaining value in weeks 3 and 4 than any of the other groups. While the percent increase in abdominal endurance for the electrical stimulation group averaged 128%, the group performing volitional exercise in conjunction with electrical stimulation increased 144% (no significant difference between the two groups).

SOURCE: Alon G, McCombe SA, Koutsantonis S, et al: Comparison of the effects of electrical stimulation and exercise on abdominal musculature. *J Orthop Sports Phys Ther* 8:567–573, 1987.

PROCEDURE 2–18

Electrical Stimulation to Increase Strength of the Triceps Surae

Parameters	Settings
Pulse duration	200 μs
Current amplitude	40–45 mA
Frequency	50 Hz (for group 1)
	2500 Hz (for group 2)
On-time	5 seconds
Off-time	50 seconds for week 1
	30 seconds for week 2
	20 seconds for week 3
Treatment duration	Fifteen contractions per day in week 1
	Twenty contractions per day in week 2
	Twenty-five contractions per day in week 3
Electrode configuration	*Proximal:* stainless-steel electrodes (45 × 55 mm) covered with wet foam rubber were placed proximally on the medial gastrocnemius close to the popliteal fossa
	Distally: on the medial gastrocnemius close to the musculotendinous junction

Electrical stimulation to increase
strength of the gastrocnemius
and soleus

Patient position	90° knee flexion with 10° ankle dorsiflexion

(continued)

PROCEDURE 2–18

Continued

OUTCOME: Thirty-six male patients, 20–23 years of age, were randomly divided into one of three groups: electrical stimulation at 50 Hz, electrical stimulation at 2500 Hz, and no electrical stimulation. After 21 days of electrical stimulation, a 50% increase in gastrocnemius strength was demonstrated using an electronic dynamometer. Both the low and high frequency electrical stimulation produced an increase in strength with no significant difference between the two outcomes. Differences in the increase of maximum isometric force between the control group and the group receiving low frequency electrical stimulation was highly significant ($P = 0.001$), as was that between the control group and those receiving high frequency electrical stimulation for 21 days ($P = 0.001$). Interestingly, a crossover training effect took place with the contralateral limb of each patient receiving electrical stimulation demonstrating an increase in strength, which remained significantly more than the negligible change in strength noted for the control group. The calf girth measurements did not significantly change for either of the legs in the control group over the 21 day period. Likewise, there was no significant change in the calf girth of the contralateral calf in either of the electrical stimulation groups, despite the crossover effect for strength. There was, however, a highly significant increase in girth (1.5–3%) of the calf after 21 days of low frequency electrical stimulation ($P < 0.01$) and a significant increase in girth of the calf receiving high frequency electrical stimulation ($P < 0.05$).

SOURCE: Cabric M, Appell JH: Effect of electrical stimulation of high and low frequency on maximum isometric force and some morphological characteristics in man. *Int J Sports Med* 8:256–260, 1987.

References

Currier DP: Neuromuscular stimulation for improving muscular strength and blood flow, and influencing changes, in *Clinical Electrotherapy*, 2d ed, Nelson RM, Currier DP (eds.). Norwalk, CT, Appleton & Lange, 1991, p 177.

Currier DP, Lehman J, Lightfoot P: Electrical stimulation in exercise of the quadriceps femoris muscle. *Phys Ther* 59(12):1508–1512, 1979.

Currier DP, Mann R: Muscular strength development by electrical stimulation in healthy individuals. *Phys Ther* 63:915–921, 1983.

Grove-Lainey C, Walmsley RP, Andrew GM: Effectiveness of exercise alone versus exercise plus electrical stimulation in strengthening the quadriceps muscle. *Physiother Can* 35:5–11, 1983.

Hosking GP, Young A, Dubowitz V, Edwards RHT: Tests of skeletal muscle function in children. *Arch Dis Child* 53:224–229, 1978.

Kloth L: Interference current, in *Clinical Electrotherapy*, RM Nelson, DP Currier(eds.). Norwalk, CT, Appleton & Lange, 1987, pp 183–207.

Kloth LC: Electrotherapeutic alternatives for the treatment of pain, in MR Gersh, *Electrotherapy in Rehabilitation*, Philadelphia, FA Davis, 1992, p 204.

Kots YM: Electrostimulation. Paper presented at the Canadian-Soviet Exchange Symposium on Electrostimulation of Skeletal Muscle. Concordia University, Montreal, December 6–10, 1977.

Kramer JF, Semple JE: Comparison of selected strengthening techniques for normal quadriceps. *Physiother Can* 35:300–304, 1983.

Kubiak RJ, Whitman KM, Johnston RM: Changes in quadriceps femoris muscle strength using isometric exercise versus electrical stimulation. *J Orthop Sports Phys Ther* 8:537–541, 1987.

Laughman RK, Youdas JW, Garrett TR, Chao EYS: Strength changes in the normal quadriceps femoris muscle as a result of electrical stimulation. *Phys Ther* 63:494–499, 1983.

Lieber RL, Silva PD, Daniel DM: Equal effectiveness of electrical and volitional strength training for quadriceps femoris muscles after anterior cruciate ligament surgery. *J Orthop Res* 14(1):131–138, 1996.

McMiken DF, Todd-Smith M, Thompson C: Strengthening of human quadriceps muscles by cutaneous electrical stimulation. *Scand J Rehabil Med* 15:25–28, 1983.

Packman-Braun R: Relationship between functional electrical stimulation duty cycle and fatigue in wrist extensor muscles of patients with hemiparesis. *Phys Ther* 68(1):51–56, 1988.

Santiesteban AJ: Physical agents and musculoskeletal pain, in *Orthopaedic and Sports Physical Therapy*, 2d ed, JA Gould (ed.). St Louis, Mosby, 1990, p 186.

Selkowitz DM: Improvement in isometric strength of the quadriceps femoris muscle after training with electrical stimulation. *Phys Ther* 65:186–196, 1985.

Selkowitz DM: High frequency electrical stimulation in muscle strengthening: A review and discussion. *Am J Sports Med* 17(1):103–111, 1989.

Selkowitz DM: Electrical currents, in *Physical Agents in Rehabilitation from Research to Practice*, MH Cameron, Philadelphia, WB Saunders, 1999; p 377.

Sisk TD, Stralka SW, Deering MB, Griffin JW: Effects of electrical stimulation on quadriceps strength after reconstructive surgery of the anterior cruciate ligament. *Am J Sports Med* 15:215–219, 1987.

Snyder-Mackler L, Garrett M, Roberts M: A comparison of torque generating capabilities of three different electrical stimulating currents. *J Ortho Sports Phys Ther* 10:297–301, 1989.

CHAPTER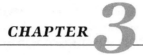

Electrical Stimulation to Enhance Bone Healing

Electrical stimulation to enhance bone healing has been reported by many clinicians and researchers. Several well-written review articles present the benefits from this form of noninvasive treatment (Connolly, 1981; Friedenberg et al 1971; Lavine and Grodzinsky, 1987). It has been demonstrated that certain electrical stimulation parameters can enhance healing, even in the cases of prolonged delayed union of bone. A delayed union is defined as no clinical or radiographic evidence of union at 4–9 months after fracture. After 9 months of no radiographic evidence of healing, the fracture is classified as a nonunion (Bassett et al, 1981).

Wolff's law states that the form and structure of bone is organized to resist perceived loads from functional demands optimally. When external forces are placed on the bone, an electrical potential is generated. Similarly, when there are no external forces on the bone, loss of bone mass occurs, as evidenced in the case of spinal cord-injured patients (Biering-Sorensen et al, 1988). The principle of cyclic loading in conjunction with electrical stimulation has been used to produce small increments of bone mass in the proximal tibia and distal femur but not in the hip of acute spinal cord-injured patients (BeDell et al, 1996).

Negative electrical potentials have been recorded at fracture sites, which follows the principle of the "current of injury" (Friedenberg and Brighton, 1966). Electrical stimulation to induce fracture healing originally used a low-amperage direct current based on the Arndt-Schultz law, which states that currents between 5 and 20 μA produce osteogenesis (Snyder-Mackler, 1995). Fukada and Yasuda (1957) suggested that the induced electrical potentials at the cathode triggered the body's piezoelectric potentials, which enhance bone repair and growth. Brighton and associates (1981) reported that 73% of nonunions healed following surgical implantation of four cathodes, each delivering 20 μA of continuous direct current for 12 weeks. While the implanted electrodes produced healing of the bone, a noninvasive method using pulsed electromagnetic fields has been proven to induce bone healing at a rate of 70–100%, depending on the simultaneous orthopedic management (Bassett, 1984; Lavine and Grodzinsky, 1987).

Pulsed electromagnetic fields (PEMFs) have been in clinical use since 1973, and the method was approved by the Food and Drug Administration in 1979 (see Figs. 3–1 and 3–2). The use of PEMFs in the presence of internal fixation (pins, screws, or a *single* plate), external fixation, or endoprostheses is not a problem since the American Society for Testing and Materials, as well as the Food and Drug Administration, now requires the use of nonmagnetic 316L steel-alloy or cobalt-chromium alloy. Pulsed electromagnetic fields (PEMFs) are an effective method of bone healing despite the presence of infection, nerve dis-

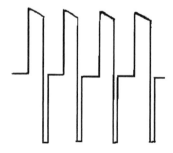

Figure 3–1 Waveform used to produce pulsed electromagnetic fields

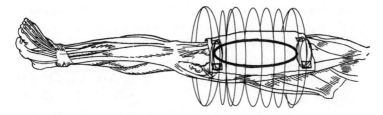

Figure 3–2   Pulsed electromagnetic field

orders, or skin defects. In addition, the length of time since the initial injury or nonunion, the patient's gender, or the age of the patient do not significantly affect the outcome of PEMFs on bone healing. Pulsed electromagnetic fields (PEMFs) have been reported to heal bone successfully in a patient with reduced bone stock following a failed total knee arthroplasty (Bigliani et al, 1983).

Pulsed electromagnetic fields (PEMFs) are generated by a time-varying current to a pair of noninvasive coils. The current creates a pulsing electromagnetic field that expands outward at right angles from the coils to penetrate the extremity (Fig. 3–2) (Skerry et al, 1991). The magnitude of the current is determined by the voltage applied to the coils by the pulse generator. Generally, the voltage generator is set between 10 and 25 V to obtain the therapeutic tissue voltage of 1–1.5 mV, depending on the diameter of the limb (including cast) and the intercoil distance (Bassett, 1984.)

Intercoil distances equal to or less than the coils' diameters produce reasonably uniform electromagnetic fields. The Helmholtz configuration consists of an intercoil distance that is equal to or less than the radius of a pair of circular coils. In all cases, the coils are positioned facing each other at 180° with the limb between them (Bassett, 1984).

The biologic response to PEMF is tissue specific. The pulse rate (15 Hz burst) used to treat ununited fractures increases cellular calcium, whereas the pulse rate (72 Hz single pulse) used to treat osteonecrosis decreases cellular calcium (Bassett, 1984). In addition, the type of tissue present in the bony gap responds to external forces, such as compression, tensile (distraction or bending), torque, or shearing. Tensile loads aid in the development of fibrous tissue, compressive loads stimulate the development of fibrocartilage, and shearing forces or torques may cause a synovial pseudoarthrosis (Flint et al, 1980). Since it is difficult to determine the predominance of the tissue in the bony gap, Bassett recommends a non-weight-bearing status for lower extremity lesions during the early phases (about 2 months) of PEMFs (Bassett, 1984). The lower extremity with a gap of more than 5 mm in the tibia or femur should be casted in 40° knee flexion or in an ambulatory spica cast. This will ensure that the non-weight-bearing status is maintained and that occasional heel-to-toe gait is prevented. For the ununited humerus fracture, a long-arm shoulder spica cast (axilla to midpalmar crease) with the arm parallel to the ground or the Orthofix External Skeletal Fixation (Orthofix, Verona, Italy) must be used to prevent the tensile loading, torque, or distraction of the humerus during the early phases of PEMFs (Bassett, 1984). Once radiographic evidence of calcification occurs, further use of PEMFs are not necessary. It is more beneficial for the patient to begin limited, protected axial compressive loading in order to activate the body's piezoelectric potentials, but the patient should remain on crutches for functional activities in order to avoid counterproductive forces until biomechanically sound bony strength has returned. The weight during axial loading must remain posterior of the center of gravity (i.e., through the heel and not through the metatarsal heads) (Bassett, 1971).

If after 4 months of PEMFs, there is no clear radiographic evidence of gap healing, fresh autogenous bone grafts are recommended, followed by immediate continuation of PEMFs. The use of bone grafts is also indicated when there is a synovial pseudoarthrosis or a bony gap that is greater than 1 cm or one half the diameter of the bone. For a cortical bone graft, the single pulse 72 Hz rate is used, and for a cancellous bone graft, the pulse burst at 15 Hz is used for successful bone healing with PEMFs (Bassett, 1984). Congenital pseudoarthrosis is treated with adult cancellous bone graft in 1 mm^3 chips with immobilization in a one and one half hip spica and PEMFs delivered at 15 Hz pulse burst for 12 hours a day for 6–14 months (Bassett et al, 1981; Kort et al, 1982; Sutcliffe and Goldberg, 1982). Sharrard (1984) reported delivering 1–1.5 mV per centimeter of bone using parallel electromagnetic coils with a single pulse at 75 Hz, 8–10 hours a day for 3 months following cancellous bone graft based on the management of 15 patients with tibial pseudoarthrosis. The electromagnetic field was applied through the plaster of a cast set with the knee at 45° of flexion.

Following treatment with PEMFs (Bassett et al, 1981), 87% of ununited tibial diaphysis fractures (n = 127) healed. In a double-blind multicenter study, PEMFs successfully healed 45% of tibial fractures (16–32 weeks postinjury at onset of treatment) using a 12-week regimen of PEMFs stimulation. The placebo group healing rate was only 12% (Sharrard, 1990). In a double-blind prospective randomized study, PEMFs were shown to shorten significantly the host graft junction healing time ($P < 0.001$) following bone tumor resection, provided chemotherapy was not used at the time of stimulation (Capanna et al, 1994).

Within the last 10 years, a success rate of 60–70% for bone healing with a gap of less than 2 mm has been obtained with the noninvasive use of capacitive coupled electrical stimulation (Abeed et al, 1998). Two capacitors, which store electrical charge when a voltage is applied, generate a potential difference when placed on either side of a limb. When an alternate current source is applied, the plates undergo a reverse polarity, charge and discharge process, generating an alternating current between the plates. At the plate-to-skin interface, the capacitance impedance decreases with frequencies in the kilohertz range, inducing electric fields that are effective for bone formation (Einhorn, 1995; Vresilovic et al, 1982). The capacitor plates are positioned on the skin opposite each other and held on lightly with an elastic band. For patients in a cast, holes are made in the plaster to accommodate the plates.

In a double-blind study, 6 out of 10 patients with nonunion for at least 9 months who were treated with capacitive coupling established a solid osseous union. The units, powered by a 9 V battery, delivered a continuous 5–10 V peak-to-peak sine wave at 60 kHz (Orthopak Bone Growth Stimulator, Biolectron, Hackensack, NJ). The difference in the healing rates of those treated with capacitive coupling and the control group was highly significant ($P = 0.004$) (Scott and King, 1994).

PROCEDURE 3–1

Pulsed Electromagnetic Stimulation of Patients Treated With Valgus Tibial Osteotomy for Degenerative Arthrosis of the Knee

Parameters	Settings
Current type/waveform	Pulsed electromagnetic field
Pulse/cycle duration	1.3 ms
Mode	Single voltage pulse
Electric field amplitude	3.0 ± 0.5 mV
Frequency	75 Hz
Treatment duration	8 hours/day for 60 days
Coil configuration	Two inductively coupled solenoid coils positioned outside the cast and held in position with a strap

OTHER: Stimulation began 3 days after surgical procedure.

OUTCOME: A double-blind study with 40 consecutive patients, 20 of whom received pulsed electromagnetic stimulation. The majority of the control group demonstrated only slight improvement in healing, whereas over 72% of the patients treated with pulsed electromagnetic stimulation demonstrated advanced stages of healing after 60 days. The authors concluded that electrical stimulation with pulsed electromagnetic fields is capable of enhancing the rate of union of a tibial osteotomy in humans.

SOURCE: Mammi GI, Rocchi R, Cadossi R, et al: The electrical stimulation of tibial osteotomies: Double-blind study. *Clin Orthop Rel Res* 288:246–253, 1993.

PROCEDURE 3-2

Treatment of Nonunions of the Proximal Fifth Metatarsal With Pulsed Electromagnetic Fields

Parameters	Settings
Current type/waveform	Pulsed electromagnetic field
Current amplitude	Magnitude of induced electric field was proportional to the rate of change
Ramp up	Increasing phase (0–20 gauss) of 200 μs
Ramp down	20 μs
Frequency of burst	15 Hz
On-time (burst duration)	4.5 ms pulse train (20 pulses)
Off-time (interburst interval)	5 μs
Treatment duration	8–10 hours/day × 2–8 months (average 4.5 months)
Coil configuration	Looped copper wire coils in formed plastic were positioned over the lateral base of the fifth metatarsal

Pulsed electromagnetic field through a cast in the treatment of nonunion of the fifth metatarsal

OTHER: Acute fractures treated with a non-weight-bearing cast for 6 weeks in conjunction with PEMFs. Weight-bearing or postoperative shoe allowed for delayed unions or nonunions.

(continued)

PROCEDURE 3–2

Continued

OUTCOME: Nine patients (average age 36 years) presented with Jones fractures at 1–5 months postinjury and were treated with pulsed electromagnetic fields.

CONCLUSION: PEMFs provided healing within an average of 18 weeks,
which, according to the author, is comparable to the healing time
frame reported in the literature for a non-weight-bearing cast
(14.8 weeks) or operative treatment (12–16 weeks).

SOURCE: Holmes GB: Treatment of delayed unions and nonunions of the proximal fifth
metatarsal with pulsed electromagnetic fields. *Foot Ankle Int* 15(10):552–556, 1994.

PROCEDURE 3–3

Treatment of Tibial Diaphyseal Delayed Unions and Nonunions With Pulsed Electromagnetic Fields Through a Non-weight-bearing Cast

Parameters	Settings
Current type/waveform	Pulsed electromagnetic field
Current amplitude	10 V of current applied to the coils to create a 2 gauss field inducing a voltage drop along the axis of the bone of 1–1.5 mV/cm.
	Heating effect was only 0.001°C from a field strength of 10^{-10} watts per square centimeter
Treatment duration	10 hours/day × 2–22 months (average 5.2 months)
Cast immobilization	*Long cast* (40° flexion) average duration = 4 months
	Short cast average duration = 1.5 months
	If fixed equinus deformity: heel of cast is thicker to ensure that axial compression exercises exert force only through heel
Coil configuration	Intercoil distance of 0.6 cm. Coils should be exactly opposite each other and parallel

Treatment of tibial diaphyseal delayed unions and nonunions through a cast using pulsed electromagnetic fields

(continued)

PROCEDURE 3–3

Continued

Parameters	Settings
Internal hardware	Screws, wires, nails, or plates made of 316L stainless steel or cobalt-chromium alloys are not removed since these components are compatible with electromagnetic fields
Axial compression exercises (non-weight-bearing stage)	*If transverse fracture with radiographic evidence of advanced healing at 1–3 months:* Patient is instructed to strike casted heel on a bathroom scale to 25–30 pounds × 50 repetitions (or as tolerated without bone ache) three times daily × 3 weeks. Progress to twice the poundage × 50 repetitions, 3 times daily × 3 weeks. Progress to partial weight-bearing
	If oblique or comminuted fracture: Patient is instructed to strike casted heel on a bathroom scale to 10–15 pounds × 50 repetitions (or as tolerated without bone ache) three times daily × 3 weeks. Progress to 20–30 pounds × 50 repetitions, 3 times daily × 3 weeks. Progress to partial weight-bearing
Patient exclusions	Synovial pseudoarthrosis with fluid-filled gap, uncontrollable motion, radiographic gap of more than 1 cm, patient noncompliance with strict non-weight-bearing status for 6 weeks
Unit	Bi-Osteogen System 204 Electro-Biology, Inc (EBI) 300 Fairfield Rd Fairfield NJ 07006

PROCEDURE 3–3

Continued

Parameters	Settings

OUTCOME: A total of 127 delayed unions and nonunions of the tibial diaphysis with histories of multiple surgical failures, present or past infections, or both were treated with pulsed electromagnetic fields. In 82% of the patients with active infection, the drainage changed from purulent to serosanguineous to serous, and then stopped within 3–5 weeks after the coils were applied. The overall success rate for osseous healing was 87%, which is comparable to surgical intervention.

SOURCE: Bassett CAL, Mitchell SN, Gaston SR: Treatment of ununited tibial diaphyseal fractures with pulsing electromagnetic fields. *JBJS* 63-A(4):511–523, 1981.

PROCEDURE 3–4

Pulsed Electromagnetic Fields for Successful Union of Chronic Pseudoarthrosis in Children

Parameters	Settings
Current type/waveform	Pulsed electromagnetic fields
Current amplitude	110 V of current applied to the coils to create a 2 gauss field inducing a voltage drop along the axis of the bone of 1–2 mV/cm of bone
Peak induced current density	10 μA
Pulse duration	300 μs
Frequency	75 Hz
Duty cycle	5:1
Treatment duration	12–16 hours/day for a minimum of 3–6 months
Cast immobilization	Long leg cast, fiberglass shell splint
Coil configuration	Two coils facing each other

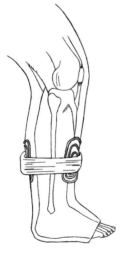

A nonoperative salvage of pseudo-arthroses and nonunions in children using pulsed electromagnetic fields

PROCEDURE 3–4

Continued

Parameters	Settings
Unit	ElectroBiology, Inc P.O. Box 21 Garfield, NJ 02026

OUTCOME: Twelve children, 6 months to 17 years of age with an average duration of congenital pseudoarthrosis of 4.9 years, were enrolled in the study. Of these, 73% experienced functional union after 20 electromagnetic sessions. In addition, 14 patients, with acquired pseudoarthroses for an average of 2.3 years, received electromagnetic field stimulation and experienced a 76% success rate in achieving union.

SOURCE: Bassett C, Pilla A, Pawluk R: A non-operative salvage of surgically-resistant pseudoarthroses and nonunions by pulsing electromagnetic fields: A preliminary report. Clin Orthop 124:128–143, 1977.

PROCEDURE 3–5

Treatment of Loosened Cemented Hip Prostheses With Pulsed Electromagnetic Fields to Postpone Revision Surgery

Parameters	Settings
Current type/waveform	Pulsed electromagnetic fields
Current amplitude	20 mV (10 μA/cm² in tissue)
Ramp up	Increasing phase (0–20 gauss) of 200 μs
Ramp down	20 μs
Frequency of burst	15 Hz
On-time (burst duration)	5 ms pulse train (25 pulses)
Off-time (interburst interval)	5 μs
Treatment duration	8 hours/day while sleeping × 6 months
Unit	Stimetics 3000 BGS Medical Englewood, CA

OUTCOME: Double-blind study with 53% of the patients (average age 65 years) who received PEMFs for 6 months demonstrating a Harris hip score greater than or equal to 80 points (prior to PEMFs the Harris hip score was 56 ± 14). In the event that the initial Harris hip score was greater than 70, an increase of at least 10 points after PEMFs was used to determine success. The Harris hip score difference between the control group and those receiving PEMFs was significant (P < 0.05). There was no correlation between the increase in hip score and the type of loosened component. While there was no osteolysis development during the period of time PEMFs was used, there was also no evidence of osteogenic refixation of the implants. By an average of 10 months after cessation of the 8 hour/day PEMFs, 60% of the patients experienced a relapse to a lower Harris hip score. The authors adapted the protocol to include a maintenance treatment of 1 hour/day of PEMFs,

PROCEDURE 3–5

Continued

which was initiated about 14 months following cessation of the 6 month 8 hours/day regimen. Despite the maintenance hour per day of PEMFs, there was no significant difference between the control group and the PEMFs group at 3 years.

CONCLUSION: PEMFs are a treatment option to delay hip revision surgery. Further study is needed to determine if additional daily hours of maintenance PEMFs or an extension of the 8 hours/day regimen would improve the outcome.

SOURCE: Kennedy WF, Roberts CG, Zuege RC, Dicus WT: Use of pulsed electromagnetic fields in treatment of loosened cemented hip prostheses: A double-blind trial. *Clin Orthop Rel Res* 286:198–205, 1993.

PROCEDURE 3–6

Capacitively Coupled Electrical Stimulation to Promote Bone Formation in Athletes With Lower Extremity Stress Fractures

Parameters	Settings
Current type/waveform	Biphasic, sinusoidal
Current amplitude	5–10 mA (using 3–6.3 V)
Frequency	60 kHz
Treatment duration	60 days for navicular fractures, 28 days for base of fifth metatarsal, 80 days for Jones fractures (navicular and fifth metatarsal)
Electrode configuration	Sticky hydrogel electrodes placed on the skin on either side of the fracture

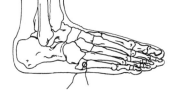

Capacitively coupled electrical stimulation to promote bone formation in athletes with stress fractures

Unit	Biolectron New Hackensack, NJ

OUTCOME: Twenty-one athletes with an average age of 21.8 years presented with a total of 25 stress fractures. Cast immobilization for 15–30 days was needed for some navicular fractures due to pain. Radiographic analysis showed that 88% of the stress fractures healed, two improved, and one did not heal. The three stress fractures that did not completely heal were located at the fifth metatarsal.

SOURCE: Benazzo F, Mosconi M, Beccarisi G, Galli U: Use of capacitive coupled electric fields in stress fractures in athletes. *Clin Orthop Rel Res* 310:145–149, 1995.

PROCEDURE 3-7

Treatment of Recalcitrant Non-unions With Capacitively Coupled Electric Field

Parameters	Settings
Current type/waveform	Biphasic, symmetrical sinusoidal
Current amplitude	5 V (7.1–10.5 mA at skin level)
Frequency	60 kHz
Treatment duration	12–40 weeks
Capacitor plate configuration	Two (3 cm diameter) stainless-steel capacitor plates placed on the skin through windows cut in opposite sides of the cast at the level of the nonunion; electrode gel applied daily under the plates

Capacitively coupled electrical stimulation in the treatment of recalcitrant nonunions

OTHER: The gel allows both a displacement current and a conducted current to pass by the skin; thus, the term *capacitive coupling* is used for the electrical method described, despite the fact that a conductive current does not exist in the system.

OUTCOME: Twenty patients with an average age of 38 years were treated with capacitively coupled electrical fields. The duration for nonunion prior to treatment ranged from 11 months to almost 15 years. Seventeen

(continued)

PROCEDURE 3–7

Continued

of the nonunions were labeled recalcitrant, meaning that they had failed to heal after either previous bone grafting, another type of electrical stimulation, or both. Of these 17 patients, four had osteomyelitis, with one actively draining nonunion site when electrical stimulation was started. A total of 77.3% of the nonunions achieved solid osseous union with no significant difference in the incidence of healing between the recalcitrant and routine nonunions. Weight-bearing on the casted lower extremity during the course of capacitive coupling treatment did not affect the result. Seventy-five percent of the patients with osteomyelitis, including the one with a draining nonunion site, healed. The presence of intramedullary rod, screws, Steinmann pins, or other forms of metal at the nonunion site at the time of capacitively coupled electrical stimulation did not affect the results.

SOURCE: Brighton CT, Pollack SR: Treatment of recalcitrant nonunion with a capacitively coupled electric field: A preliminary report. *JBJS* 67-A(4):577–585, 1985.

PROCEDURE 3–8

Capacitively Coupled Electrical Stimulation for Treatment of Failed Long Bone Fractures

Parameters	Settings
Current type/waveform	Biphasic symmetrical sine wave
Current amplitude	6 V
Frequency	63 kHz
Treatment duration	7–8 hours/day for an average of 15 weeks
Capacitor plate configuration	Two 40 mm nonmagnetic stainless-steel capacitor plates positioned on the skin opposite to each other, less than 80 mm apart, and held on lightly with an elastic band. For patients wearing a plaster cast, holes were made in the cast to accommodate the plates

Capacitively coupled electrical stimulation in the treatment of failed long bone fracture unions

OUTCOME: Sixteen patients, 17–56 years of age, with nonunion of long bone fractures (ranging from 9 months to 6.3 years in duration) were enrolled in the study. All patients presented with a radiographic gap of less than 2 mm. Sixty-nine percent achieved full consolidation of the fracture within an average of 19 weeks, 15 of which included application of electrical stimulation.

SOURCE: Abeed RI, Naseer M, Abel EW: Capacitively coupled electrical stimulation treatment: Results from patients with failed long bone fracture unions. *J Orthop Trauma* 12(7):510–513, 1998.

References

Abeed RI, Naseer, Abel EW: Capacitively coupled electrical stimulation treatment: Results from patients with failed long bone fracture unions. *J Orthop Trauma* 12(7):510–513, 1998.

Bassett CAL: Biophysical principles affecting bone structure, in *The Biochemistry and Physiology of Bone*, Vol III, GH Bourne (ed). New York, Academic Press, 1971.

Bassett CAL: The development and application of pulsed electromagnetic fields (PEMFs) for ununited fractures and arthrodeses. Symposium on Electrically Induced Osteogenesis. *Orthop Clin North Am* 15(1):61–87, 1984.

Bassett CAL, Caulo M, Kort J: Congenital "pseudoarthroses" of the tibia: Treatment with pulsing electromagnetic fields. *Clin Orthop* 154:136–149, 1981.

Bassett CA, Mitchell SN, Gaston SR: Treatment of ununited tibial diaphyseal fractures with pulsing electromagnetic fields. *JBJS* 63-A(4):511–523, 1981.

BeDell KK, Scremin AME, Perell KL, Kunkel CF: Effects of functional electrical stimulation-induced lower extremity cycling on bone density of spinal cord-injured patients. *Am J Phys Med Rehabil* 75:29–34, 1996.

Biering-Sorensen F, Bohr H, Schaadt O: Bone mineral content of the lumbar spine and lower extremities years after spinal cord lesion. *Paraplegia* 26:293–301, 1988.

Bigliani LU, Rosenwasser MP, Caulo N, et al: The use of pulsing electromagnetic fields to achieve arthrodesis of the knee following failed total knee arthroplasty: A preliminary report. *JBJS* 65-A:480–485, 1983.

Braddom RL: *Physical Medicine and Rehabilitation*, Philadelphia, WB Saunders, 1996, p. 483.

Brighton CT, Black J, Friedenberg ZB, et al: A multicenter study of the treatment of non-union with constant direct current. *JBJS* 63-A:2–13, 1981.

Capanna R, Donati D, Masetti C, et al: Effect of electromagnetic fields on patients undergoing massive bone graft following bone tumor resection: A double-blind study. *Clin Orthop Rel Res* 306:213–221, 1994.

Connolly JF: Selection, evaluation and indications for electrical stimulation of ununited fractures. *Clin Orthop Rel Res* 161:39–53, 1981.

Einhorn TA: Current concepts review: Enhancement of fracture healing. *JBJS* 77-A:940–956, 1995.

Flint MH, Gillard GC, Merrilees MJ: The effect of local physical environmental factors on connective tissue organization and glycosaminoglycan synthesis, in *Fibrous Proteins: Scientific, Industrial and Medical Aspects*, 2d ed, DAD Parry, LK Creamer (eds.): London, Academic Press, 1980; pp 107–119.

Friedenberg ZB, Brighton CT: Bioelectric potentials in bone. *JBJS* 48-A: 915–923, 1966.

Friedenberg ZB, Harlow MC, Brighton CT: Healing of nonunion of the medial malleolus by means of direct current: A case study. *J Trauma* 11:883–885, 1971.

Fukada E, Yasuda I: On the piezoelectric effect of bone. *J Phys Soc Japan* 10:1158–1169, 1957.

Kort JK, Schink MM, Mitchell SN, et al: Congenital pseudoarthrosis of the tibia: Treatment with pulsing electromagnetic fields. *Clin Orthop* 165:124–137, 1982.

Lavine LS, Grodzinsky AJ: Current concepts review: Electrical stimulation of repair of bone. *JBJS* 69-A:626–630, 1987.

Scott G, King JB: A prospective, double-blind trial of electrical capacitive coupling in the treatment of non-union of long bones. *JBJS* 76A: 820–826, 1994.

Sharrard WJ: Treatment of congenital and infantile pseudoarthrosis of the tibia with pulsing electromagnetic fields. *Orthop Clin North Am* 15(1):143–162, 1984.

Sharrard WJW: A double-blind trial of pulsed electromagnetic fields for delayed union of tibial fractures. *JBJS* 72-B(3):347–355, 1990.

Skerry TM, Pead MJ, Lanyon LE: Modulation of bone loss during disuse by pulsed electromagnetic fields. *J Orthop Res* 9:600–608, 1991.

Snyder-Mackler L: Electrical stimulation for tissue repair, in AJ Robinson, L Snyder-Mackler, *Clinical Electrophysiology: Electrotherapy and Electrophysiologic Testing*. Baltimore, Williams & Wilkins, 1995; p 323.

Sutcliffe ML, Goldberg AAJ: The treatment of congenital pseudoarthrosis of the tibia with pulsing electromagnetic fields: A survey of 52 cases. *Clin Orthop* 166:45–57, 1982.

Vresilovic E, Pollack ST, Brighton CT: A generalised theoretical approach to the determination of local field parameters during capacitively coupled electrical stimulation *in vivo*. *Trans Bioelect Repair Growth Soc* 2:10, 1982.

CHAPTER 4

Electrical Stimulation to Enhance Circulation

The use of electrical stimulation to improve circulation or reduce edema has been studied by few investigators despite the rapid improvements noted clinically. The effectiveness of high voltage pulsed current to reduce edema, once considered a well-established protocol, has not withstood the criteria of significant improvement once studied in a scientific manner (Griffin et al, 1990; Michlovitz et al, 1988). Unfortunately, many of the protocols used in the clinics and presented in this chapter have not been included in controlled research studies. Clearly, more scientific research is needed to prove the significance of these treatments if funding from third-party payers is expected.

While not all of the protocols specifically list the polarity or the location of the anode or cathode, the following guidelines are the most popular recommendations.

General Guidelines

Acute Edema

In the case of sensory level electrical stimulation or high voltage pulsed current, place the anode over the site of injury. This form of sensory stimulation (about 100 pps) requires the use of the anode over the site, a positive polarity, or both, and is reserved for use in the acute stage (minutes after injury to no more than 48 hours after injury).

Chronic Edema

Muscle contraction and relaxation creates a pumping action that has been shown to resolve edema once it is formed. This form of motor level electrical stimulation (about 20 pps) requires the use of the cathode over the site of edema, a negative polarity, or both.

PROCEDURE 4–1

Sensory Level Electrical Stimulation for Acute Edema Control

Parameters	Setting
Current type/waveform	Monophasic pulsed current
Pulse duration	20–100 μs
Current amplitude	10% below motor threshold
Frequency	120 pps
Treatment duration	30 minutes every 4 hours
Electrode configuration	Small cathode over the injured area, dispersive anode over remote site

Electrical stimulation to reduce acute edema

Polarity	Negative

OUTCOME IF TREATED ONLY ONCE A DAY: Grade II ankle sprain treated 4 hours postinjury for only 30 minutes daily resulted in a 30% reduction in swelling within 24 hours. Over the next 5 days, electrical stimulation once a day resulted in temporary reduction in swelling with a 50% return rate within the 24 hour period.

SOURCES:

Hooker DN: Electrical stimulating currents, in WE Prentice, *Therapeutic Modalities for Allied Health Professionals.* New York, McGraw-Hill, 1998; p 112.

Selkowitz DM: Electrical currents, in MH Cameron, *Physical Agents in Rehabilitation from Research to Practice,* Philadelphia, WB Saunders, 1999; p 396.

PROCEDURE 4–2

Sensory Level Electrical Stimulation for Acute Edema Control of Sprained Ankle

Parameters	Settings
Current type/waveform	Monophasic pulsed current or high voltage pulsed current
Pulse duration	2–50 µs
Current amplitude	Below motor threshold (~30–50 V)
Frequency	120 pps
Treatment duration	30 minutes every 4 hours
Electrode configuration	Two carbon-rubber electrodes submerged in cold water bath next to ankle. If using a whirlpool for submersion, tape electrodes to side of whirlpool to prevent them from becoming entangled in the agitator

Underwater electrical stimulation to reduce acute edema in the sprained ankle

Polarity	Negative

OTHER: Instruct the patient to keep the foot fully submerged during the treatment. When ending the treatment, turn the stimulator off first, then the whirlpool.

OUTCOME: No research reported to support parameters.

SOURCE: Snyder-Mackler L: Electrical stimulation for tissue repair, in Clinical Electrophysiology: Electrotherapy and Electrophysiologic Testing, 2d ed, AJ Robinson, L Snyder-Mackler, (eds.). Baltimore, Williams & Wilkins, 1995; pp 325–326.

PROCEDURE 4–3

Motor Level Electrical Stimulation for Postacute Edema Control

Parameters	Settings
Current type/waveform	Medium frequency burst alternating current (AC) (Russian stimulation)
	Medium frequency beat AC (interferential)
Cycle duration	100–600 μs
Duty cycle	50% if medium frequency burst AC
Current amplitude	Maximum tolerated contraction
Ramp up	1–2 seconds
Ramp down	1–2 seconds
Frequency	30–50 bursts per second
On-time	2–10 seconds
Off-time	2–10 seconds
Treatment duration	15–60 minutes
	Over motor nerves of innervated muscles that will cause muscle contraction at desired area

Motor level electrical stimulation
to control postacute edema

SOURCE: Selkowitz DM: Electrical currents, in MH Cameron, *Physical Agents in Rehabilitation from Research to Practice.* Philadelphia, WB Saunders, 1999; p 398.

PROCEDURE 4–4

Motor Level Electrical Stimulation of the Agonist and Antagonist Muscles for Edema Control

Parameters	Settings
Current type/waveform	Monophasic high voltage pulsed current (HVPC) *or* symmetrical biphasic pulsed current (BPC) *or* asymmetrical biphasic pulsed current (BPC)
Pulse duration if BPC	200–500 µs
Pulse duration if HVPC	20–100 µs
Modulation	Reciprocal or intermittent
Current amplitude	Maximum tolerated contraction
Frequency	> 60 pps
On-time	5 seconds
Off-time	5 seconds
Treatment duration	20–30 minutes
Electrode configuration	Cathode (–) over edematous area

SOURCE: Hecox B, Mehreteab TA, Weisberg J: *Physical Agents: A Comprehensive Text for Physical Therapists.* Norwalk, CT, Appleton & Lange, 1994; p 290.

PROCEDURE 4–5

Electrical Stimulation to Reduce Acute Edema Due to Local Hematoma, Bursitis, or Hemarthroses

Parameters	Settings
Current type/waveform	Symmetrical biphasic pulsed current
Mode	Synchronous channel stimulation
Pulse duration	300–500 μs
Current amplitude	Sensory only
Ramp up	3 seconds
Ramp down	3 seconds
Frequency	> 80 pps
On-time	10 seconds
Off-time	10 seconds
Treatment duration	20–30 minutes, one to two times per day
Electrode configuration	Cathode (–) over edematous area

OUTCOME: No research reported to support parameters.

SOURCE: Stralka S: Protocol for the treatment of edema, in *LOGIX Guidelines*. St. Paul, MN, EMPI, 1987.

PROCEDURE 4–6

Electrical Stimulation to Reduce Chronic Edema Due to Venous Insufficiency or Lymphatic Obstruction

Parameters	Settings
Current type/waveform	Symmetrical biphasic pulsed current
Mode	Alternating channel stimulation
Pulse duration	300–500 μs
Current amplitude	Maximum tolerated, but < 100 mA
Ramp up	3 seconds
Ramp down	2 seconds
Frequency	50–80 pps
On-time	15 seconds
Off-time	5 seconds
Treatment duration	15–60 minutes two to four times per day
Electrode configuration	Target muscle groups of edematous limb or reciprocal stimulation of agonist and antagonist

SOURCE: Stralka S: Protocol for the treatment of edema, in *LOGIX Guidelines*. St. Paul, MN, EMPI, 1987.

PROCEDURE 4–7

Use of Garment Electrode With Electrical Stimulation to Reduce Edema in the Distal Limb

Parameters	Settings
Current type/waveform	Symmetrical biphasic pulsed current
Pulse duration	300 μs
Current amplitude	Motor stimulation
Frequency	50 pps
Treatment duration	20–30 minutes/ day
Electrode configuration	Target agonist and antagonist of muscle groups for the digits of the edematous limb. Glove is the anode. The cathodes of the stimulator are separately connected to 4 × 3 cm karaya-padded carbon rubber electrodes placed over the dorsal and volar surfaces of the forearm proximal to the wrist and at least 2 cm from the mesh glove (anode)

Mesh glove electrode to reduce edema in the hand

Unit	Respond II EMPI (Formerly sold by Medtronic) 599 Cardigan Road St. Paul, MN 55126 (800) 328–2536
Mesh glove	Prizm-Medical 3400 Corporate Way Duluth, GA 30096

(continued)

PROCEDURE 4–7
Continued

Parameters	Settings
Gloves, socks, knee, elbow, and garment electrodes	BioMedical Life-Systems P.O. Box 1360 Vista, CA 92083-1360 (800) 726-8367

NOTE: This protocol was reported for use on hemiplegic patients, but it has been used clinically in the reduction of edema in orthopedic and neurologic patients, including those with reflex sympathetic dystrophy. To date, there are no peer-reviewed articles that identify the ideal parameters for edema reduction using the glove; thus, the values originally reported by Dimitrijević and associates are reported here.

SOURCES:

Dimitrijević MM, Stoki DS, Wawro AW, Wun CC: Modification of motor control of wrist extension by mesh-glove electrical afferent stimulation in stroke patients. *Arch Phys Med Rehabil* 77(3):252–258, 1996.

Dimitrijević MM: Mesh-glove. 1. A method for whole-hand electrical stimulation in upper motor neuron dysfunction. *Scand J Rehabil Med* 26:183–186, 1994.

Dimitrijević MM: Mesh-glove. 2. Modulation of residual upper limb motor control after stroke with whole-hand electric stimulation. *Scand J Rehabil Med* 26:187–190, 1994.

PROCEDURE 4–8

Motor Level Electrical Stimulation in Conjunction with Low-dose Heparin to Prevent Deep Vein Thrombosis (DVT) in Spinal Cord-injured Patients

Parameters	Settings
Current type/waveform	Biphasic pulsed current
Pulse duration	50 μs
Duty cycle	33%
Frequency	10 pps for contractions five times per minute
On-time	4 seconds
Off-time	8 seconds
Treatment duration	23 hours for 28 days
Electrode configuration	Two channels: Channel one over motor points of tibialis anterior and channel two over motor points of the gastrocnemius for simultaneous stimulation
	A second unit with two channels needed for identical configuration on opposite leg

Prevention of deep vein thrombosis (DVT) after acute spinal cord injury

Unit	Myocare Stimulator (Number 6280) 3M 3M Center Building 304-1-0 St. Paul, MN 55144-1000

(continued)

PROCEDURE 4-8

Continued

OUTCOME: Forty-eight patients, less than 2 weeks postinjury, were randomly assigned to three groups: one of which received the above electrical stimulation protocol with 5000 units of heparin subcutaneously every 8 hours. The incidence of DVT was 8 out of 17 in the placebo group, 8 out of 16 in the heparin group, and 1 out of 15 in the electrical stimulation and heparin group.

CONCLUSION: Deep vein thrombosis (DVT) after acute spinal cord injury is best prevented by decreasing both hypercoagulability and stasis through the combination of low dose heparin and the use of prophylactic electrical stimulation to the lower extremities.

SOURCES:

Jacobs SR, Jaweed MM, Herbison GJ, Stillwell GK: Electrical stimulation of muscle, in *Therapeutic Electricity and Ultraviolet Radiation*, 3d ed., GK Stillwell (ed.). Baltimore, Williams & Wilkins, 1983; pp 124–173.

Lindstrom B, Korsan-Bengstonk J, Jonsson O, et al: Electrically-induced short-lasting tetanus of calf muscles for prevention of deep vein thrombosis. *Br J Surg* 69:203–206, 1982.

Merli GJ, Herbison GJ, Ditunno JF, et al: Deep vein thrombosis: Prophylaxis in acute spinal cord-injured patients. *Arch Phys Med Rehabil* 69:661–664, 1988.

Rosenberg IL, Evans M, Pollock AV: Prophylaxis of postoperative leg vein thrombosis by low dose subcutaneous heparin or perioperative calf muscle stimulation: A controlled clinical trial. *Br Med J* 1:649–651, 1975.

PROCEDURE 4-9

Motor Level Electrical Stimulation to Increase Vasodilation for the Treatment of Raynaud's Disease or Diabetic Polyneuropathy

Parameters	Settings
Current type/waveform	Balanced asymmetrical biphasic pulsed current
Current amplitude	Motor response
Frequency	100 pps
Treatment duration	30 minutes
Electrode configuration	Over motor nerves of innervated muscles

SOURCE: Kaada B: Vasodilation induced by transcutaneous nerve stimulation in peripheral ischemia: Raynaud's phenomenon and diabetic polyneuropathy. *Eur Heart J* 3:303–314, 1982.

PROCEDURE 4–10

Motor Level Electrical Stimulation to Increase Circulation Treatment of Acrocyanosis in Tetraplegia

Parameters	Settings
Current type/waveform	Balanced asymmetrical biphasic pulsed current
Pulse duration	350 µs
Current amplitude	Motor response
Frequency	30 pps
Treatment duration	30–40 minutes, one to three times per week for 6 weeks
Electrode configuration	Over motor nerves of innervated muscles (quadriceps if treating cyanotic feet)

Electrical stimulation to increase circulation in tetraplegic spinal cord-injured patients with acrocyanosis and ulcers of the feet

OUTCOME: After 5 weeks of electrical stimulation, the discoloration in feet disappeared, and the ulcers were nearly healed.

SOURCE: Twist DJ: Acrocyanosis in a spinal cord-injured patient: Effects of computer controlled neuromuscular electrical stimulation: A case report. *Phys Ther* 70:45–49, 1990.

PROCEDURE 4–11

Sensory Level Electrical Stimulation to Improve Circulation

Parameters	Settings
Current type/waveform	Medium frequency burst AC (Russian stimulation)
	Medium frequency beat AC (interferential)
Cycle duration	20–100 μs
Duty cycle	50% if medium frequency burst AC
Current amplitude	Maximum tolerated tingling
Frequency	50–200 bursts per second
Modulation	Optional
Treatment duration	20–60 minutes
Electrode configuration	Over sensory nerves

OUTCOME: No research reported to support parameters.

SOURCE: Selkowitz DM: Electrical currents, in MH Cameron, *Physical Agents in Rehabilitation from Research to Practice*, Philadelphia, WB Saunders, 1999; p 395.

References

Griffin JW, Newsome LS, Stralda SW, Wright PE: Reduction of chronic post-traumatic hand edema: A comparison of high voltage pulsed current, intermittent pneumatic compression, and placebo treatments. *Phys Ther* 70:279–286, 1990.

Michlovitz S, Smith W, Watkins M: Ice and high voltage pulsed stimulation in treatment of lateral ankle sprains. *Orthop Sports Phys Ther* 9:301–304, 1988.

CHAPTER 5

Electrical Stimulation to Promote Wound Healing

Intact skin has an electrical potential difference with the epidermis being negative in relation to the dermis. Wounded skin demonstrates the existence of a natural bioelectric current called the *current of injury*, in which the wound and adjacent epidermis become positively charged in relation to the uninjured tissue for 24–48 hours postinjury (Becker and Murray, 1967; Jaffee and Vanable, 1984). This disruption of the normal electric potentials may trigger the healing process. As healing progresses, the wound becomes increasingly negative through the proliferative stage with a wound closure rate of 1 mm per day. When healing is complete (approximately 8–9 days postinjury), the epidermis returns to its normal negatively charged state in relation to the dermis.

Direct current electrical stimulation with the anode over the wound attracts neutrophilic leukocytes and macrophages, while the low amperage direct current at the cathode attracts fibroblasts (Dunn et al, 1988; Orida and Feldman, 1988). In addition, cathodal stimulation has been used to increase the strength and density of surgical scars (Assimacopoulos, 1968; Konikoff, 1976).

To avoid disrupting the granulation tissue of a healing wound, many researchers propose applying electrical stimulation through the existing wound dressing. One study compared the conductance properties of

wound dressings and reported that saline-soaked gauze, hydrated algi-
nates, and hydrogels were excellent conductors (Selkowitz et al, 1998).
Bactericidal agents, such as Betadine, hydrogen peroxide, chlorhexi-
dine, and Dakin's solution, are cytotoxic and retard the growth of granulation tissue (Becker and Spadaro, 1978; Higgins and Ashry, 1995).
While there are many published reports on the effectiveness of the
use of electrical stimulation for wound healing, it is difficult to determine the most effective protocol since researchers report on a variety
of currents (high voltage pulsed current, low voltage electrical stimulation, biphasic pulsed current, monophasic pulsed current, direct cur-
rent, low intensity direct current, low intensity stimulation, micro-
amperage, or microcurrent). Reviewing the medical reports from the
past decade can be confusing due to the changes in the accepted terminology for electrotherapy currents. For instance, galvanic stimulation
is no longer used to describe direct current (*Electrotherapeutic Terminology in Physical Therapy,* 1990). In addition, the preferred term for
high voltage pulsed current is now monophasic pulsed current. Similarly, low intensity stimulation was once called microcurrent electrical
neuromuscular stimulation (MENS) and was later referred to as microcurrent electrical stimulation (MES) or microamperage stimulation
(MS). Low intensity stimulation (LIS) is now the preferred term for
stimulation using less than 1 mA. While low intensity direct current
(LIDC) falls into the category for classification of LIS, the acronym
LIDC is still used (Hooker, 1998).

   The clinician, when choosing electrotherapy to aid in wound healing, must take into consideration the polarity of stimulation (order and
timing of switching polarity), the electrode wire type (silver effect on
healing), the use of bacteriocidal or cytotoxic agents, the type of infec-
tious agent (*Pseudomonas aeruginosa. Escherichia coli, Staphylococcus
aureus*, no bacteria, etc), the wound etiology (burn, surgical incision,
venous statis ulcer, pressure sore, etc), the stage of healing (acute,
chronic, proliferative, etc), and the age and health status of the patient.
If the clinician is using a published article for the basis of the electrotherapy protocol, it is important to note if additional interventions
were provided before or in conjunction with electrotherapy that might
aid or hinder the healing rate. Furthermore, laboratory animals, such as
pigs, rabbits, dogs, hamsters, and rats, are often used for studies on heal-

ing rates; however, these animals all heal significantly differently than humans.

In vitro studies and experiments with rats and rabbits have demonstrated that the use of low intensity direct current or low amplitude current using the cathode for stimulation is bactericidal (Barranco and Berger, 1974; Rowley, 1972; Rowley et al, 1974). The use of monophasic pulsed current (previously referred to as high voltage pulsed current) for bactericidal effects has been proposed based on an in vitro study; however, the voltage and exposure times are too high to use safely on humans (Kincaid and Lavoie, 1989). Many vendors propose electrical parameters for human use that have only been reported in the literature through animal studies. It is up to the clinician to verify each protocol and read the referenced article prior to applying the electric current to the patient.

Prior to treating the wound of a patient, the clinician should read the laboratory reports for the results of a recent culture of the wound. The presence of an infection or the organism in the wound will affect the treatment plan. Reusable electrodes and sponges should be disinfected prior to use by soaking for 20 minutes in two-thirds of an ounce of Mikro-Quat solution per gallon of water (Ecolab, St. Paul, MN). After disinfection, the electrodes and sponges should be removed from the solution using sterile gloves. The electrodes should be rinsed thoroughly using sterile 0.9% saline or sterile water. The sponges, covered with sterile saline-soaked 4 × 4 gauze, should be secured to the electrodes (Kalinowski et al, 1996).

When in contact with the patient's body fluids, the clinician must follow the guidelines published by The Center for Disease Control for Universal Precautions (Centers for Disease Control, 1987; Centers for Disease Control, 1989).

1. Gloves should be worn when touching blood, body fluids, mucous membranes, nonintact skin of patients, or when handling items soiled with body fluids.
2. The eyes and face of the health care provider should be covered with a face shield when performing procedures likely to generate droplets of blood or body fluids. Similarly, the health care worker should be protected with moisture-resistant gowns or aprons when splashing of the patient's body fluids is probable.

3. The health care provider should wash his or her hands in running water using vigorous scrubbing for a minimum of 1 minute after removal of gloves.
4. Any skin surface of the health care worker contaminated by the patient's body fluid should be washed immediately as described in item 3.
5. A disinfectant solution, such as 10% sodium hypochlorite (bleach), should be used to clean spills of body fluid immediately after they occur.
6. All specimens, gauze, bandages, and so forth that were contaminated with the patient's body fluids should be placed in leakproof red bags or containers with secure lids. These materials should be disposed of in accordance with the policies in effect at the institution.
7. Sharp instruments should be used only when no alternative procedure is available.
8. Before leaving the area, all protective wear must be removed and discarded appropriately, and hands must be washed.

To document the effectiveness of the treatment, the perimeter and depth of the wound should be measured. The following procedure is one of many methods of documenting wound healing.

Don mask and sterile gloves. Explain the procedure to the patient. The depth of the wound should be measured by inserting the tip of a sterile cotton-tipped applicator into the wound. Place a gloved fingernail on the wooden applicator that is level with the edge of the epidermis. Remove the applicator, and measure the distance in millimeters from the cotton tip to the gloved fingernail on the wooden applicator. Measure the width and shape of the wound by holding a transparency page a set distance from the patient's skin. Using a permanent marker, trace the outline of the wound. Do not lie the transparency page on the patient's skin. This method allows direct comparison of the size of the wound by overlaying the transparency pages or by using different colored markers on the same transparency page.

Once the wound care has been completed, documentation of the treatment should include measurement of the wound perimeter, depth of the wound, type of microorganism present (if any), general characteristics of the wound, medications, type of dressings, and the electrical stimulation parameters. Many clinicians will photograph the wound from a set distance or trace the wound outline onto a transparent sheet as a record of the healing process.

If using direct current, the electrodes should be configured so that the current densities do not exceed 0.1–0.5 mA per square centimeter. The current density is the amount of current flow per cubic volume. To decrease the current density, decrease the frequency or increase the intrapulse interval. The amplitude is generally less than 5 mA, and the treatment duration is less than 15 minutes (Robinson, 1995). The dispersive pad should be four times larger than the treatment electrode. Clean the dispersive pad well with soap and water. An area of intact skin at least 12 inches from the wound site should be cleansed with alcohol prior to application of the dispersive pad. The dispersive pad may be on the back, shoulder, abdomen, or opposite thigh (Hooker, 1998).

PROCEDURE 5–1

Monophasic Pulsed Current for Wound Healing

Parameters	Settings
Current type/waveform	Monophasic pulsed current, twin spike, which is also called high voltage pulsed current
Pulse duration	20–100 μs
Current amplitude	100–200 V
Frequency	50–200 pps
Treatment duration	30–120 minutes, 3 to 4 times a day, 5 ×/week, 1–8 weeks
Electrode configuration	Smaller treatment electrode over wound, dispersive electrode at remote site

Wound care using monophasic pulsed current (i.e., high voltage pulsed current)

Polarity	Initially positive

SOURCE: Selkowitz DM: Electrical currents, in MH Cameron, *Physical Agents in Rehabilitation from Research to Practice*. Philadelphia, WB Saunders, 1999; p 401.

PROCEDURE 5–2

Monophasic Pulsed Current for Wound Healing

Parameters	Settings
Current type/waveform	Monophasic pulsed current, twin spike, which is also called high voltage pulsed current
Pulse duration	20–100 µs
Current amplitude	150 V (750 mA)
Frequency	50 pps
Treatment duration	30–120 minutes 4 to 3 times a day, 5 times a week for 8 weeks
Electrode configuration	Aluminum foil electrode over wound, dispersive electrode proximal to wound

Treatment of a previously non-responsive heel wound using an aluminum foil electrode

Polarity	Negative
After day six:	
Current amplitude	100 V (500 mA)
Frequency	80 pps
Polarity	Positive

OTHER: Mechanically debrided as needed.

(continued)

PROCEDURE 5–2

Continued

OUTCOME: After an average of 11 weeks, 154 geriatric patients from 11 facilities experienced healing in almost 90% of their wounds. These wounds were previously nonresponsive to traditional nursing care for an average of 2.4 months prior to electrical stimulation.

SOURCE: Unger PG: A randomized clinical trial of the effect of HVPC on wound healing. *Phys Ther* 71(6):S118, 1991.

PROCEDURE 5–3

Monophasic Pulsed Current for Treatment of Chronic Stage III or IV Skin Ulcer

Parameters	Settings
Current type/waveform	Monophasic pulsed current
Current amplitude	30–35 mA
Frequency	128 pps
Treatment duration	30 minutes b.i.d. with 4–8 hours between treatments for 4 weeks
Electrode configuration	Saline-soaked gauze into wound covered by 7.5 × 7.5 cm sponge electrode. A 16 × 16 cm dispersive electrode moistened with water was placed a minimum of 30.5 cm from the wound

Treatment of stage III or IV chronic ulcer with saline soaked gauze and sponge electrode

Polarity	Initially negative; changed to positive after wound was debrided or drained and was alternated every 3 days thereafter
Unit	Vara/Pulse
	TGS Electronics
	5 Ladd Road
	New Gisborne 3438
	Australia

OTHER: Surgical or whirlpool debridement received for 10% of the participants.

Continued for Stage II—see Procedure 5–4.

PROCEDURE 5–4

Monophasic Pulsed Current for Treatment of Chronic Stage II Skin Ulcer Healing

Parameters	Settings
Current type/waveform	Monophasic pulsed current
Current amplitude	35 mA
Frequency	128 pps with negative polarity
	64 pps once a stage II ulcer
Treatment duration	30 minutes b.i.d. with 4–8 hours between treatments for 4 weeks
Electrode configuration	Saline-soaked gauze into wound covered by 7.5 × 7.5 cm sponge electrode. A 16 × 16 cm dispersive electrode moistened with water was placed a minimum of 30.5 cm from the wound

Treatment of stage II chronic ulcer with saline soaked gauze and sponge electrode

Polarity	Negative until wound debrided or drained, and then alternated every 3 days until the ulcer reached a stage II classification. When stage II, the polarity was alternated daily
Unit	Vara/Pulse TGS Electronics 5 Ladd Road New Gisborne 3438 Australia

PROCEDURE 5–4

Continued

___

OUTCOME: Forty-seven patients (average age of 64 years) participated in this multicenter, randomized, double-blind study. The average healing rate was 14% per week for the treatment group and 8.25% per week for the control group. After 4 weeks, 26 wounds in the treatment group were 44% of the original size in comparison to the control group, whose wounds were 67% of the original size. Thus, the wounds of the group treated with electrical stimulation healed significantly faster than the wounds of the control group ($P < 0.02$).

___

SOURCE: Feeder JA, Kloth LC, Gentzkow GD: Chronic dermal ulcer healing enhanced with monophasic pulsed electrical stimulation. *Phys Ther* 71(2):639–649, 1991.

PROCEDURE 5–5

Monophasic Pulsed Current for Treatment of Chronic Stage III Wounds

Parameters	Settings
Current type/waveform	Monophasic pulsed current
Pulse duration	140 µs
Current amplitude	30, 35, or 40 mA*
	If infected, use 35 mA
Frequency	64 or 128 pps*
	If infected, use 128 pps
Treatment duration	30 minutes twice a day (4–8 hours apart) for 14 weeks
Electrode configuration	Saline-soaked gauze electrode over wound; dispersive pad 12 inches from wound

Electrical stimulation of a stage III wound that has been present over 3 months

Polarity	Positive or negative, depending on protocol*

PROCEDURE 5–5

Continued

Parameters	Settings
Contraindications	Patients excluded if wounds near eye or larynx, if wounds covered by eschar, if major blood vessel hemorrhaging, or if patient is cancerous, has peripheral vascular problems, clots, phlebitis, active osteomyelitis, diabetes mellitus, extreme obesity, cardiovascular disease, is pregnant, has a pacemaker, or is on long-term steroid therapy, chemotherapy, or radiation therapy
Unit	Dermapulse Wound Management System Staodyn, Inc. 1225 Ken Pratt Blvd Longmont CO 80502-1379

OTHER: Podiatrist conducting study received a grant from Staodyn, Inc.

OUTCOME: Multicenter study of 26 stage III wounds that had been present for an average of 3.4 months. The wounds, 4–100 cm^2 in diameter, included pressure ulcers, vascular lesions, and surgical wounds that extended into the muscle. Ninety-two percent of the patients showed a good to excellent response after 2 weeks of electrical stimulation.

SOURCE: Mulder GD: Treatment of open-skin wounds with electrical stimulation. *Arch Phys Med Rehabil* 72:375–377, 1991.

*Choice of amplitude, frequency, and polarity were not described by author in any further detail.

PROCEDURE 5–6

High Voltage Pulsed Current for Treatment of Pressure Ulcers in Spinal Cord-injured Patients

Parameters	Settings
Current type/waveform	High voltage pulsed current
Interpulse interval	75 μs
Current amplitude	200 V
Frequency	100 pps
Treatment duration	1 hour/day for 20 consecutive days
Electrode configuration	Saline-soaked gauze in wound covered by heavy duty aluminum foil that was cut larger than perimeter of wound. The aluminum foil electrode, which was attached with an alligator clip cathodal (negative) lead wire, was wrapped in plastic wrap circumferentially to hold it in place. Dry gauze was taped over the site to further secure the electrode. If needed, a sandbag was placed on top. The 20 × 25 cm dispersive electrode was placed over a wet cloth on the medial thigh

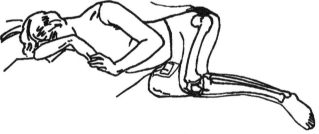

Saline-soaked gauze and aluminum foil electrode to apply electrical stimulation to a pressure ulcer located over the greater trochanter on a spinal cord-injured patient

PROCEDURE 5–6

Continued

Parameters	Settings
Polarity	Negative
Unit	Intelect 500 HVPC Stimulator
	Chattanooga Corp
	PO Box 4287
	Chattanooga, TN 37405

OTHER: Twice a day wounds were mechanically debrided (no enzymatic debridement) and covered with Cora-Klenz ointment (Carrington Labs, Dallas TX 75356)

OUTCOME: Seventeen spinal cord-injured patients with stage II, III, or IV gluteal or sacral pressure ulcers were randomly assigned to a placebo or electrical stimulation group. The digitized area of the wound was measured before treatment and then every 5 days. The patients receiving high voltage pulsed current demonstrated significant improvements in the healing rate at day 5 ($P = 0.03$), day 15 ($P = 0.05$) and day 20 ($P = 0.05$).

SOURCE: Griffin JW, Tooms RE, Mendius RA, et al: Efficacy of high voltage pulsed current for healing of pressure ulcers in patients with spinal cord injury. *Phys Ther* 71(6):433–444, 1991.

PROCEDURE 5–7

High Voltage Pulsed Current for Treatment of Stage III Lower Extremity Chronic (>8 weeks) Ulcers

Parameters	Settings
Current type/waveform	Monophasic pulsed current, twin spike, which is also called high voltage pulsed current
Pulse duration	5–8 μs
Current amplitude	250 V
Frequency	100 pps
Treatment duration	20 minutes/day, 5 days/week for 4 weeks
Electrode configuration	Smaller treatment electrode over wound, dispersive electrode at remote site
Polarity	Negative for first four treatments, then positive

OTHER: Debridement as needed, cytotoxic Betadine, whirlpool, and wet-to-dry dressings used.

OUTCOME: Twelve patients were divided between a treatment group and a control group. The average age of the treatment group was 63 years; whereas the average age for the control group was 10 years younger. Wound etiologies for 7 of the 12 wounds included venous stasis or diabetic ulcer. In the first 2 weeks, the healing rate was greater for the group treated, but at the end of the study, the authors concluded that the treatment did not significantly improve the healing rate. It is important to note that this study allowed the use of Betadine, which has been proven to be a cytotoxic hindrance to healing of wounds. In addition, a "sterile" whirlpool was used. The frequency of either of these treatment adjuncts was not clearly defined. It was also not clear how many patients or which group received these additional treatments.

SOURCES:

Gogia PP, Marques RR, Minerbo GM: Effects of high voltage galvanic stimulation on wound healing. *Ostomy/Wound Management* 38:29–35, 1992.

Selkowitz DM: Electrical currents, in MH Cameron, *Physical Agents in Rehabilitation From Research to Practice*. Philadelphia, WB Saunders, 1999.

PROCEDURE 5–8

Low Voltage Electrical Stimulation for the Treatment of Chronic Burn Wounds

Parameters	Settings
Current type/waveform	Direct current
Current amplitude	10–25 V, 10–20 mA (tingling sensation)
Treatment duration	10 minutes
Electrode configuration	Smaller treatment electrode over wound, dispersive electrode at remote site

Low voltage electrotherapy used for the treatment of chronic burn wounds

Polarity	Negative for first four treatments, then positive

OTHER: No antibiotics during treatment.

OUTCOME: Wounds were 3 months to 2 years postpartial or full thickness burns. Epithelization was observed after 3 days. Nineteen out of twenty patients achieved reduction in the size of the wounds. Some of these patients had previous skin grafts, some went on to skin grafts once the size of the wound decreased.

SOURCE: Fakhri O, Amin MA: The effect of low-voltage electric therapy on the healing of resistant skin burns. J Burn Care Rehabil 8:15–18, 1987.

PROCEDURE 5–9

Low Intensity Direct Current for the Treatment of Chronic Skin Ulcers

Parameters	Settings
Current type/waveform	Direct current
Current amplitude	300–500 µA (innervated) 500–700 µA (denervated)
Current density	30–110 µA/cm²
Treatment duration	2 hours on, 4 hours off, 5 days/week for 5 weeks
Electrode configuration	Flexible carbon gas sterilized electrodes over saline-dampened gauze packed wound
	Dispersive electrode 15–25 cm proximal to wound. When positive polarity is used at the wound site, the dispersive electrode must be at least twice the size of the active electrode

Low intensity direct current
used for the treatment of chronic
skin ulcers

Polarity	Negative for first three treatments, then positive over the wound until it healed or a plateau in healing was noted. If plateau was reached, the protocol of negative polarity at the wound site for a 3 day period was restarted

PROCEDURE 5–9

Continued

Parameters	Settings
Unit	Prototype parts supplied by AGAR, Kibbutz Ginosar, Israel 14980

OTHER: All wounds were debrided prior to beginning study. The treatment group did not require further debridement. Control group debrided as often as every 2 weeks. A few patients received Dakin's solution or Betadine, which is now known to affect healing adversely (Selkowitz, 1999). It was unclear from reading the article to which group these patients belonged. Four control patients received whirlpool treatments four to five times per week.

OUTCOME: Thirty patients (average age more than 70 years of age) with sacral or below knee ulcers were matched on age, wound etiology, and size. The average duration of the wounds was 8.6 months (treatment group) and 5.2 months (control). While there was no statistical difference in the wound healing between the treatment and control groups in the first 2 weeks of the study, significant differences were noted after the third week. Note that the control group was debrided as much as every 2 weeks, whereas the treatment group was not debrided during the period of electrical stimulation. The healing rate in the treatment group was reported to be 1.5–2.5 times faster than the healing rate of the control group.

SOURCES:

Carley PJ, Wainapel SF: Electrotherapy for acceleration of wound healing: Low intensity direct current. *Arch Phys Med Rehabil* 66:443–446, 1985.

Selkowitz DM: Electrical currents, in MH Cameron, *Physical Agents in Rehabilitation from Research to Practice*. Philadelphia, WB Saunders, 1999.

RE 5-10

Low Intensity Direct Current for Healing of Ischemic Skin Ulcers: Preliminary Study

Parameters	Settings
Current type/waveform	Direct current
Current amplitude	600 µA for 2 hours, then observe the wound. If serous, then the amplitude is too low. Increase to 800 µA, and apply for 2 hours. If the wound is bloody, the amplitude is too high. Decrease to 400 µA, and following a 4 hour period, reapply at the lower amplitude for 2 hours
Treatment duration	2 hours on, 4 hours off, 3 times a day × 18 months
Electrode configuration	2 × 2 inch copper mesh cathode (replaced every 2 weeks) sandwiched between six layers of dry sterile gauze and then saturated with Ringer's or saline solution before being placed over wound; anode sandwiched between four layers of sterile gauze and saturated in Ringer's or saline solution before being placed 15 cm proximal to the lesion

Low intensity direct current used for the treatment of ischemic skin ulcers

Polarity	Cathode stimulation over wound for 3 days
	If infection: negative electrode over wound until infection-free

PROCEDURE 5-10

Continued

Parameters	Settings
	followed by 3 additional days of cathodal stimulation; then switch electrodes so that anode (positive electrode) is over *If no infection:* switch electrodes so that anode is over the wound. Once plateau in healing is noted, switch electrodes so that cathode (negative electrode) is over wound for 3 days. At this point, the final healing stage is entered, and polarity should be switched every 24 hours

OTHER: Wounds were debrided daily followed by scrubbing of the raw base with PHisoHex. The use of PHisoHex is no longer recommended due to its cytotoxic properties as reported by Selkowitz.

OUTCOME: Clinicians studied 67 patients with 75 ischemic skin ulcers. After 18 months of daily electrical stimulation, 40% of the wounds had completely healed.

SOURCES:

Selkowitz DM: Electrical currents, in *Physical Agents in Rehabilitation from Research to Practice.* Philadelphia, WB Saunders, 1999; p 399.

Wolcott LE, Wheeler PC, Hardwicke HM, Rowley BA: Accelerated healing of skin ulcers by electrotherapy: Preliminary clinical results. *South Med J* 62:795–801, 1969.

PROCEDURE 5–11

Low Intensity Direct Current for Healing of Ischemic Skin Ulcers: Second Study

Parameters	Settings
Current type/waveform	Direct current
Current amplitude	200–400 µA if intact sensation 400–800 µA for chronic wounds
Treatment duration	2 hours on/4 hours off 3 times a day, daily for an average of 5 weeks (up to 24 weeks)
Electrode configuration	Each electrode is sandwiched between four layers of saline-soaked gauze
Polarity	Negative electrode (cathode) over wound with anode 15 cm proximal to wound for 3 days
	If infection: keep the negative electrode over wound until infection clears, followed by an additional 3 days; then the positive electrode over the wound with the negative electrode 15 cm distal to the wound
	If no infection: switch electrodes so that anode over wound with cathode 15 cm distal to wound (note that the positive electrode is always proximal, and the negative electrode is distal)

PROCEDURE 5-11

Continued

Parameters	Settings
Unit	Tri-tonics Lab, Inc 1004 Pamela Dr. Euless, TX 76039 Vitron/Ritter Sybron Corp PO Box 848 Rochester, NY 14603

OUTCOME: The study enrolled 67 patients with 106 ischemic skin ulcers (one present for 36 years). The mean healing rate (28.4% reduction in size per week) of the ulcers treated with electrical stimulation was twice as fast as the healing rate for the control group (14.7% reduction in size per week).

SOURCE: Gault WR, Gatens PF: Use of low intensity direct current in management of ischemic skin ulcers. *Phys Ther* 56(1):265–269, 1976.

References

Assimacopoulos D: Wound healing promotion by the use of negative electric current. *Am Surg* 34:423–431, 1968.

Barranco S, Berger T: In vitro effect of weak direct current on *Staphylococcus aureus*. *Clin Orthop* 100:250–257, 1974.

Becker RO, Murray DG: Method for producing cellular dedifferentiation by means of very small electrical currents. *Trans NY Acad Sci* 29:606, 1967.

Becker RO, Spadaro JA: Treatment of orthopedic infections with electrically generated silver ions: A preliminary report. *JBJS* 60-A:871–881, 1978.

Centers for Disease Control: Recommendations for prevention of HIV transmission in health-care settings. *MMWR* (Suppl) 36:3S, 1987.

Centers for Disease Control: Guidelines for prevention of transmission of human immunodeficiency virus and hepatitis B virus to health-care and public-safety workers. *MMWR* 38:1, 1989.

Dunn MG, Doillon CJ, Berg RA, et al: Wound healing using a collagen matrix: Effect of DC electrical stimulation. *J Biomed Mater Res: Applied Biomechanics* 22:191–206, 1988.

Electrotherapeutic Terminology in Physical Therapy, Section on Clinical Electrophysiology. Alexandria, Virginia, American Physical Therapy Association, 1990.

Higgins KR, Ashry HR: Wound dressings and topical agents. *Clin Podiatr Med Surg* 12:31–40, 1995.

Hooker DN: Electrical stimulating currents, in WE Prentice, *Therapeutic Modalities for Allied Health Professionals*. New York, McGraw-Hill, 1998; p 109.

Jaffee LF, Vanable JW Jr: Electric fields and wound healing. *Clin Dermatol* 2:34–44, 1984.

Kalinowski DP, Brogan MS, Sleeper MD: A practical technique for disinfecting electrical stimulation apparatuses used in wound treatment. *Phys Ther* 76(12):1340–1347, 1996.

Kincaid CB, Lavoie KH: Inhibition of bacterial growth in vitro following stimulation with high voltage, monophasic pulsed current. *Phys Ther* 69:651–655, 1989.

Konikoff JJ: Electrical promotion of soft tissue repairs. *Ann Biomed Eng* 4:1–5, 1976.

Orida N, Feldman JD: Directional protrusive pseudopodial activity and motility in macrophages induced by extracellular electric fields. *Cell Motility* 2:243–255, 1988.

Robinson AJ: Instrumentation for electrotherapy, in AJ Robinson, L Snyder-Mackler, *Clinical Electrophysiology: Electrotherapy and Electrophysiological Testing*, 2d. ed. Baltimore, Williams & Wilkins, 1995; p 73.

Rowley B: Electrical current effects of *Escherichia coli* growth rates. *Proc Soc Exp Biol Med* 139:929–934, 1972.

Rowley B, McKenna J, Chase G, et al: The influence of electrical current on an infecting microorganism in wounds. *Ann NY Acad Sci* 238:543–551, 1974.

Selkowitz DM, Cameron M, Wain P, et al: Electrical conductance of wound dressings used in the treatment of full-thickness wounds. Combined Sections Meeting, APTA, Boston, February 1998.

CHAPTER 6

Nerve Conduction Velocity

Nerve conduction studies are carried out by electrical stimulation of a nerve fiber and recording the resultant action potential from a muscle supplied by the nerve fiber or from a more proximal or distal segment of the nerve fiber. When stimulation or recording can be carried out at two separate nerve sites, the conduction time between the two nerve sites can be measured in milliseconds. Figure 6–1 illustrates the muscle action potential, recorded from the muscle fibers, following stimulation of the motor axons.

Orthodromic is defined as the signal in the motor axons traveling in the natural direction of the motor nerve signal (ie., from the spinal cord to the myoneural junction and then to the extrafusal muscle fibers). In contrast, orthodromic for a sensory nerve would naturally travel from the distal point of stimulation to the spinal cord. The sensory nerve signal is recorded in the microvolt range (1000 times smaller than the motor nerve signal), and, thus, requires use of the signal averaging technique. (*Antidromic* is defined as the signal traveling in the direction opposite of what would naturally be expected. For example, the antidromic signal in the motor axon travels from the muscle fibers to the spinal cord.)

Electrical stimulation at site 1 will elicit an orthodromic muscle action potential. The conduction time from the stimulus artifact (S) to the initial deflection of the action potential is called the distal latency (Ld). Electrical stimulation of site 2 on the nerve fibers will generate

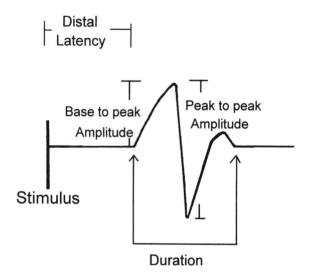

Figure 6–1   Action potential velocity recorded from the muscle following stimulation to the axon

another muscle action potential with a more prolonged latency (Lp). See Figure 6–2.

To calculate the nerve conduction velocity, the distance between the two nerve stimulation sites must be measured in millimeters. The difference between the latency time at the second stimulation site and the distal latency is calculated. The distance is then divided by the latency difference using the following formula:

$$\text{Nerve conduction velocity } (m/s) = \frac{D \text{ (in mm)}}{Lp - Ld \text{ (in ms)}}$$

Electrical muscle and nerve signals are very small in amplitude and can sometimes be masked by electrical noise, movements, external electromagnetic and radio wave signals, or dirty electrodes or skin. The recording electrode must be clean with no breaks in its recording surface or the connecting wires. Careful preparation of the skin at the recording sites with water, alcohol, or both will help obtain a clear signal. Slight abrasion of the skin with fine grade sandpaper may improve the recording signal by producing a lower skin impedance.

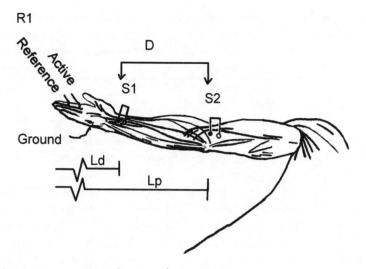

Figure 6–2   Nerve conduction velocity measure

Application of the active recording electrode on the motor point of the muscle or on the skin on top of the nerve fibers will result in a better recording signal. In denervated muscle, the motor point will not be located in the usual place. Application of the reference recording electrode on a nearby, less active site, such as the joint, bony prominence, or tendon, will result in a monopolar recording with a clearly identifiable signal. (Monopolar recording is recording from a single active site in reference to a less active site, whereas bipolar recording involves both the active and reference electrodes recording electrical signals from the muscle or nerve.) The ground electrode should be applied to a less active site between the stimulation and recording electrodes. This placement will reduce the effect of the stimulus artifact on the recorded potential and will produce a straight baseline with identifiable deflection of the action potential.

Use the appropriate amplification sensitivity/gain. A sensitivity/gain that is too high will result in an increasingly large and possibly clipped signal (a signal cut at the top or the bottom of the action potential). A sensitivity/gain that is too low will result in a smaller signal that is not identifiable.

Use the appropriate filter setting to obtain a nondistorted signal. The low pass and high pass filters pass electrical signals that are contained in such a bandwidth. It will cut off all other signals below or above the filter setting. When the filter setting for the high pass (that passes the high frequency signal) is set too high, the low frequency components of the signal will be cut off, causing a peaked action potential. When the filter setting for the low pass (that passes the lower frequency signal) is set too low, the action potential will lose the high frequency components. This setting will result in a smaller, more rounded appearance for the action potential.

The appropriate sweep speed of the electromyograph (EMG) unit is crucial for recording a clinically valid signal. The action potential must be clearly visible in the middle of the oscilloscope (display screen) of the EMG unit. Faster or slower sweep speeds will result in an action potential at the far ends of the screen with no identifiable shape. In this case, it would be inaccurate to measure the duration of the action potential.

Electrical stimulation, using a constant current at about 1 pps, should begin at a minimal intensity and gradually increase until there is no more increase in the amplitude of the action potential. Submaximal stimulation may not activate all of the nerve fibers, resulting in a delayed action potential and erroneous calculation of the conduction velocity for the nerve.

Parameters of Nerve Conduction Studies

The Stimulus Artifact

The electrical stimulus (reported as intensity), delivered by the electric stimulator, is recorded by the active electrode and presented as a vertical line at the far left aspect of the display screen. The duration of the artifact is dependent on the duration of the electrical stimulus. The latency measurement is taken from the beginning of the vertical line representing the stimulus artifact.

The Distal Latency

The time delay from the beginning of the stimulus artifact to the first deflection of the action potential is called the distal latency or the latency to deflection (Fig. 6–1). Distal motor latency for motor nerve conduction studies includes (1) the conduction time in the nerve segment from the stimulation site to the myoneural junction, (2) the signal transmission through the myoneural junction, and (3) the conduction time in the muscle fibers. Because of the different value of conduction in these three segments, the distal latency cannot be used to calculate the conduction velocity.

The distal latency may be a useful parameter for detecting mononeuropathy or polyneuropathy. Distal latency is prolonged in patients with polyneuropathies due to demyelination of large diameter nerve fibers of the distal nerve. The distal latency is also useful in detecting entrapment neuropathies since demyelination of the entrapped nerve segment causes prolongation of the distal latency. To detect prolonged distal latencies, a comparison is made of the distal latency for a 10 cm segment of the suspected nerve to the distal latency for a 10 cm segment of another nerve.

The Amplitude of the Action Potential

The amplitude of the action potential (peak-to-peak or baseline-to-peak) reflects the number of axons that have been activated (Fig. 6–1). The amplitude of the action potential is decreased significantly in the case of nerve entrapment. The amplitude of the compound action potential varies between subjects for the same nerve, making comparisons within a population of patients inaccurate.

The Action Potential Waveform

The compound action potential shape reflects the degree of synchronization of motor unit activity. If the number of phases of the action potential increase, there may be reduced synchronization of the motor units during a muscle contraction. This finding is seen in patients with regenerating nerve fibers or advanced carpal tunnel syndrome, or in older subjects. (Sabbahi and Sedgwick, 1982). On the other hand, action potential polyphasia and reduced motor unit synchronization might be due to degeneration of some nerve axons with resultant collateral sprouting of other nerve axons. The newly sprouted replacement axons have a slower conduction velocity, and, thus, a late contribution to the compound action potential. Another cause of poor synchronization of the compound action potential is local demyelination. Varying degrees of demyelination might cause slower conduction velocity of the activated axons.

The duration of the compound action potential is the amount of time from the first deflection (deviation above or below the isoelectric baseline) to its return to the baseline. It is affected by the distance between the two recording electrodes.

The Proximal Latency

The proximal latency is the conduction time from the more proximal nerve site to the contracted muscle. Electrical stimulation of the median nerve at the elbow or the axilla will produce proximal latency of two different values (elbow-to-abductor pollicis brevis and axilla-to-abductor pollicis brevis). It is useful to detect nerve damage at the more proximal sites.

The Conduction Time

The conduction time is the time taken by the electric pulse to travel to a specific nerve segment. The distal latency may be measured followed by the testing of the proximal latency. In both distal and proximal latencies, a delay at the myoneural junction or a slower conduction of the muscle fibers will reduce the value for the conduction velocity. Therefore, subtraction of the distal from the proximal latency would result in the conduction time. The conduction time might be shorter in larger diameter fibers for the same length of nerve fibers. In patients with demyelination or entrapment neuropathies, the conduction time would be prolonged.

The Conduction Velocity

The conduction velocity is the speed at which a nerve fiber may conduct an electric signal. It reflects the functional performance of the nerve fibers. Some nerve fibers, such as the Ia sensory afferents, conduct signals faster than others, such as the alpha or gamma motor fibers. Information that requires prompt response of the central nervous system travels via fast conducting large diameter nerve fibers.

Conduction velocities are positively correlated with the diameter of nerve fibers. The conduction velocity of large nerve fibers is faster than that of small diameter nerve fibers. For this reason, the conduction velocity of the sensory nerves is faster than that of the motor nerves.

In addition, nerve fibers in the upper extremities have a higher value of the conduction velocity than the lower extremities. In long nerves, the conduction velocity usually becomes slightly faster as the nerve fiber diameter becomes bigger toward the proximal segment of the nerve. Myelinated nerve fibers conduct signals significantly faster than the nonmyelinated nerve fibers.

Placement of the Stimulating and Recording Electrodes

Electrical stimulation electrodes should be applied accurately on the skin overlying the nerve to be stimulated. Slight displacement of the stimulation electrode will require a higher stimulus intensity and produce a noxious sensation for the patient.

The orientation of the active cathode in relation to the reference anode electrodes is of technical importance. In monopolar stimulation, the active cathode electrode is applied on the nerve while the anode is applied on the opposite side of the limb. In bipolar stimulation, the active cathode, where the depolarization of the axonal membrane begins, should be positioned ahead of the reference electrode and toward the target. In motor conduction studies, the target is the muscle, and the cathode should be applied distal to the reference electrode. In orthodromic sensory nerve conduction studies, the target is the site of the recording electrode on the nerve fiber, and the cathode should be applied proximal to the anode. In H-reflex and F-wave studies, the target is the spinal cord, and the cathode should be positioned more proximal to the reference electrode.

The active recording electrode should be applied on the muscle belly (motor point) of the tested muscle. This is where the largest action potential can be recorded. Displacement of the active electrode from the motor point will result in significant exponential reduction of the recorded compound action potential. The reference electrode should be applied at a less active site (in monopolar recording) or on an active site of the nerve or muscle (in bipolar recording). The ground electrode should always be placed on a less active site (a bony site if possible) between the stimulation and recording electrodes. This will reduce the effect of the stimulus artifact on the recorded potentials.

Factors Affecting the Accuracy of Nerve Conduction Studies

Factors that affect nerve conduction accuracy include the following:

• Temperature of the skin and the core temperature are important factors affecting the values of the conduction studies. Lower skin temperature may cause an increased conduction time, prolong the distal latency, and reduce the value of the conduction velocity. Most clinicians prefer the skin to be 32°C or 90°F prior to nerve conduction testing.
• If there is no clear deflection of the compound action potential, incorrect calculation of the conduction velocity may occur.
• An error in measuring the correct distance between the two sites of the stimulation electrodes may result in incorrect calculation of the conduction velocity.
• Older subjects have a slower value of conduction velocity, as well as a smaller amplitude of the evoked action potentials as compared to the younger population.
• Broken electrode wires.
• Dirty electrodes or an old, scratched electrode surface.
• Fluorescent lights or activation of an automatic electronic dimmer.
• Electromagnetic equipment operating close to the EMG room.
• Electric drill in operation or ungrounded power tool in operation.
• Radio frequency signal from TV, radio, and pagers.
• Inappropriate location or a small or not properly connected ground electrode.
• Recording and stimulation cables crossing each other.
• Incorrect connection to the preamplifier or amplifier.
• Movement of the electrode wires.
• Electrode gel bridging between electrodes.
• Excessive perspiration of the patient causing changing skin impedance.
• Excessive movement of the patient during electric stimulation.
• Use of a transcutaneous electrical nerve stimulation (TENS) machine during stimulation and recording.
• Anomalies of innervation.

Anomalies of innervation may result in abnormal electrophysiologic measurements. For example, abnormal anastomosis between the median and the ulnar nerves at the upper segment of the forearm may result in a small amplitude compound action potential recorded at the abductor digiti minimi (ADM) if the stimulation is proximal to the anastomosis, whereas stimulation of the ulnar nerve distal to the anastomosis will result in normal potentials in the ADM. Stimulation of the median nerve below the anastomosis level will show no action potentials in the ADM.

Other anomalies might involve collateral innervation of the ADM muscle from a branch in the median nerve at the level of the forearm in up to 13% of normal subjects. These anomalies may cause some difficult decisions, especially in patients with forearm and hand pathologies.

Median Nerve Conduction Study

Anatomic Considerations

The median nerve is a mixed nerve that originates from the C6–T1 spinal nerve roots and the lateral and medial cords of the brachial plexus. It is most superficial at the cubital fossa and the anterior aspect of the wrist. It supplies mainly the anterior compartment of the forearm and the thenar muscle group. It supplies cutaneous sensation to the lateral two thirds of the anterior aspect of the palm and the lateral $3\frac{1}{2}$ fingers, including the dorsal surface of the terminal phalanges. Cutaneous sensation of the middle finger is supplied by the C7 nerve root.

The cutaneous sensation of the index and the thumb is supplied by C6 or C7 nerve roots. The median nerve gives rise to a pure motor branch at the forearm called the anterior interosseous nerve that supplies the anterior forearm muscles.

Common Sites of Injury to the Median Nerve

Common median nerve injury sites are

- the plexus level at the shoulder girdle,
- the cubital fossa between the two heads of the pronator teres, and
- the wrist, such as in cases of carpal tunnel syndrome.

Median (Motor) Nerve Conduction Study

Electromyograph (EMG) Set-up

Sensitivity/gain: 2–5 mV/div
Filter setting: 10 Hz–2 kHz
Sweep speed: 3–5 ms/div

Patient Position (Fig. 6–3)

The patient is positioned supine with arm at 45° abduction, supinated, with the wrist in a neutral position.

Recording Electrode Placement (Fig. 6–4)

Active (black) electrode: on motor point of abductor pollicis brevis
Reference (red) electrode: on the metacarpophalangeal joint
Ground (green) electrode: on back of the hand

Stimulation Sites (Fig. 6–4)

First site (S1):   anterior to the wrist 10 cm proximal to the active recording electrode

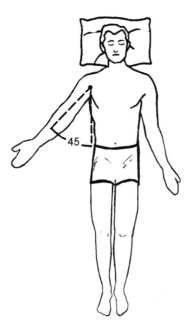

Figure 6–3 Patient position for median or ulnar nerve conduction study

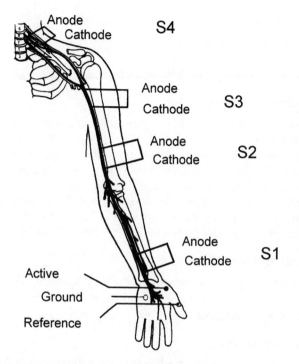

Figure 6–4   Median (motor) nerve conduction study

Second site (S2):   at the cubital fossa medial to the biceps tendon or
                    between the biceps and brachialis muscles
Third site (S3):   at the medial upper one quarter of the arm (between
                    the biceps and triceps muscles)
Fourth site (S4):   above the medial one third of the clavicle and lateral to
                    the sternomastoid muscle (Erb's point)

Always apply the active electrode (cathode/black) distal to the reference
(anode/red) with a 2 cm difference between the two electrodes.

Stimulation Parameters

Stimulus duration: 0.1 ms
Stimulation rate: 1 pps
Stimulus intensity: supramaximal for the motor action potentials

Supramaximal stimulation can be obtained with increasing stimulus
intensity that generates maximum action potential, then increasing the
stimulus intensity a little higher.

Normal Values

Distal latency:	3–5 ms
Amplitude:	3–15 mV
Conduction velocity:	> 50 meters/second

Technical Comments

1. Avoid the jugular vein when applying electrical stimulation above the clavicle.
2. Use constant current stimulation as it is more comfortable.
3. Shape of recorded action potentials should be similar at stimulation sites S1, S2, S3, and S4 of the median nerve.
4. Distance measurement of the nerve segment between the axillary site (upper arm) and Erb's point must be taken while the externally rotated shoulder is placed in a 90° angle of abduction.

Clinical Applications

Carpal tunnel syndrome, mononeuropathy, polyneuropathy, median nerve trauma, and brachial plexus injuries can all be confirmed with the use of a nerve conduction study.

Clinical Perspective

In carpal tunnel syndrome, the distal latency of the median nerve is usually prolonged when compared to the distal latency of the ulnar nerve for an equal nerve distance. In polyneuropathy, the distal latency for both nerves might be comparable.

Median Nerve (Sensory) Nerve Conduction Study

Orthodromic Technique

In recording median nerve sensory/orthodromic, the stimulation electrode ring is placed on the electrode-gel covered thumb. The recording electrode is placed at different sites, such as the wrist, cubital fossa, and upper arm.

Electromyograph (EMG) Set-up

Sensitivity/gain:	10–20 µV/div
Filter setting:	100–1000 Hz
Sweep speed:	1 ms/div

Patient Position (Fig. 6–3)

The patient is positioned supine with the arm at 45° abduction with the forearm supinated and the wrist in the neutral position.

Recording Electrode Placement

Active (black) electrode: distally placed
Reference (red) electrode: proximally placed with 2 cm between electrodes
Ground (green) electrode: on the back of the hand

Recording Sites

First recording site (R1):   on the anterior aspect of the wrist proximal to the wrist crease between the tendons for the flexor carpi radialis and palmaris longus (when present)
Second recording site (R2):   cubital fossa at the medial side to the biceps tendon or between the biceps and brachialis muscles on the medial side of the lower one quarter of forearm
Third site (R3):   medial side of the upper one quarter of the arm between the biceps and triceps muscles

Stimulating Ring Electrode Placement

STANDARD TECHNIQUE (FIG. 6–5)

Cathode: metacarpal phalangeal (MP) joint of thumb
Anode: interphalangeal (IP) joint of thumb
Ground electrode: on the back of the hand

Stimulating Ring Electrode Placement

ROTH TECHNIQUE (FIG. 6–6)

In this alternative technique the hand-held, two-prong electrical stimulation electrode may be placed between the index and middle fingers at the level of the MP and proximal interphalangeal (PIP) joints of the closely adducted fingers. The operator holds the patient's two fingers together with the two-prong hand-held electrode placed between the fingers.

Cathode: proximally placed
Anode: distally placed
Ground (green) electrode: on the back of the hand

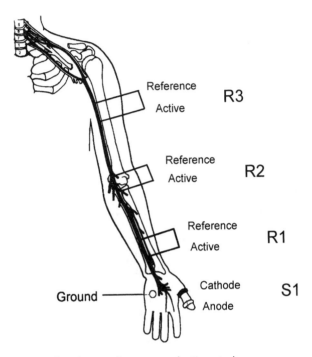

Figure 6–5 Median (sensory) nerve conduction study

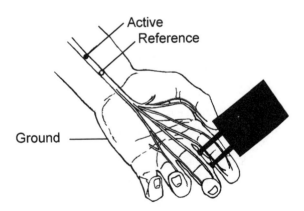

Figure 6–6 Roth technique for median (sensory) orthodromic nerve conduction study

Electrical Stimulation Parameters

Stimulus duration: 0.1 ms
Stimulation rate: 1 pps
Stimulus intensity: at threshold of maximum sensory action potential

Normal Values

Distal latency: 2.75–3.25 ms
Amplitude: 10–90 µV
Conduction velocity: > 55 meters/second

Technical Comments

Average 10 pulses while recording the action potential at the wrist level. Recording the sensory nerve potentials at the elbow and the axilla levels requires averaging more than 10 pulses (20–60 pulses). The patient's skin should be at room temperature (32°C or 90°F).

Clinical Application

Sensory nerve conduction testing is useful in diagnosing and monitoring carpal tunnel syndrome, mononeuropathy or polyneuropathy, and trauma to the median nerve.

Clinical Perspective

The distal latency of action potentials of the median nerve sensory fascicles is usually prolonged when compared to equal distance of ulnar or radial nerve sensory segments.

Median Nerve (Sensory) Antidromic Technique

To determine the nerve conduction velocity of the sensory aspect of the median nerve, the antidromic technique is used. In this procedure, the recording electrodes are taped on the digits while the stimulating electrodes are placed at the wrist, cubital fossa, or upper arm. Occasionally, the axilla is the location for the stimulation.

Electromyograph (EMG) Set-up

Sensitivity/gain: 10–20 µV/div
Filter setting: 100–1000 Hz
Sweep speed: 1 ms/div

Patient Position (Fig. 6–3)

The patient is positioned supine with the arm in 45° abduction.

Recording Electrode Placement (Fig. 6–7)

Use ring electrodes with conductive gel for recording.

Active (black) electrode: on the MP joint of the index finger
Reference (red) electrode: on the PIP joint of the index finger
Ground (green) electrode: on the back of the hand

Stimulation Sites (Fig. 6–7)

First point (S1):   anterior aspect of the wrist proximal to the wrist
                        crease and between the tendons for the flexor carpi
                        radialis and palmaris longus
Second point (S2):   cubital fossa medial to the biceps tendon *or* 2 cm
                        proximal to the medial epicondyle between the
                        biceps and brachialis muscles
Third point (S3):   medial side of the upper one quarter of the arm
                        between the biceps and triceps muscles

Electrical Stimulation Parameters

Stimulus duration: 0.1 ms
Stimulus rate: 1 pps
Stimulus intensity: to elicit maximum sensory action potential

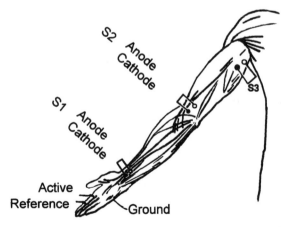

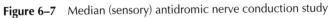

Figure 6–7   Median (sensory) antidromic nerve conduction study

Normal Values

Distal latency: 2.75–3.25 ms
Amplitude: 10–60 μV
Conduction velocity: > 55 meters/second

Technical Comments

The conduction velocity should increase in value with a more proximal nerve segment due to increased diameter of nerve fibers. Keep the patient's hand at room temperature (32°C or 90°F) throughout the testing time.

Clinical Application

Carpal tunnel syndrome, mononeuropathy and polyneuropathy, median nerve trauma, and brachial plexus injuries can all be detected using this technique.

Clinical Perspectives

The conduction velocity using the antidromic and orthodromic techniques should be comparable; however, the amplitude of the sensory compound action potential may be a little higher in the antidromic recording.

Ulnar Nerve Conduction Studies: Anatomic Considerations

The ulnar nerve originates from the C8 and T1 spinal roots. It is the continuation of the medial cord of the brachial plexus. It lies in close proximity to the median nerve at the axilla and passes behind the medial epicondyle of the humerus to the forearm. It innervates the flexor carpi ulnaris muscles, the medial portion of the flexor digitorum profundus (III and IV) in the forearm. It passes in the Guyon's canal at the wrist level to the hand. It then innervates the hypothenar muscle groups, palmar and dorsal interossei muscles, and the deep head of the flexor pollicis brevis, as well as the adductor pollicis muscle. It supplies cutaneous sensation to the medial one and one half fingers and medial side of the hand over the hypothenar muscle group.

The common sites for ulnar nerve injuries are at the medial cord of the brachial plexus, such as in cases of thoracic outlet syndrome; at the medial side of the elbow and behind the medial humeral epicondyle; or at the wrist level. The deep motor branch sometimes is subjected to injury with hand trauma.

Ulnar (Motor) Nerve Conduction Study

Electromyograph (EMG) Set-up

Sensitivity/gain: 3–5 mV/div
Filter setting: 10 Hz–2 kHz
Sweep speed: 3–5 ms/div

Patient Position (Fig. 6–8)

The patient is positioned supine with the arm at 90° abduction with a 90° elbow flexion.

Recording Electrode Placement (Fig. 6–9)

Active (black) electrode: on motor point of abductor digiti minimi
Reference (red) electrode: MP joint of little finger
Ground (green) electrode: back of the hand

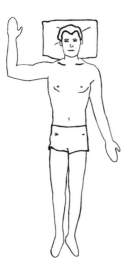

Figure 6–8 Patient position for ulnar nerve conduction study

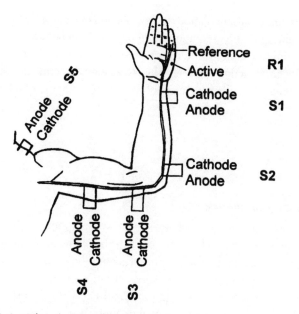

Figure 6–9   Ulnar (motor) nerve conduction study

Stimulation Sites (Fig. 6–9)

First site (S1):   anterior and medial aspect of the wrist and 10 cm
                    proximal to the active recording electrode; cathode
                    distally placed

Second site (S2):   at the medial side of the forearm 3–4 cm distal to the
                    medial epicondyle of the humerus

Third site (S3):   medial side of the arm and 4 cm proximal to the medial
                    epicondyle about 8–10 cm proximal to the second site

Fourth site (S4):   medial side of the upper one quarter of the arm
                    between the biceps and triceps muscles

Fifth site (S5):   above the medial third of the clavicle and lateral to the
                    sternocleidomastoid muscle (Erb's point)

Electrical Stimulation Parameters

Stimulus duration   0.1 ms

Stimulus rate: 1 pps

Stimulus intensity: at suprathreshold level for maximum motor action
                    potential for the ADM muscle

Supramaximal stimulation can be obtained by increasing the electrical stimulus until the maximum action potential can be recorded. A further increase in stimulus intensity would not cause any increase in the amplitude of the action potential. This is considered a supramaximal stimulation. It ensures full recruitment of all motor units in the ADM muscle.

Normal Values

Distal latency: 2.5–3.5 ms
Amplitude: 5–15 mV
Conduction velocity: > 53 meters/second

Technical Comments

The distance measurement between the stimulation sites below and above the elbow should be obtained with the elbow in 90° angle since measurement of the distance with a straight elbow would result in an erroneous lower conduction velocity. Distance measurement for the nerve segment between the upper arm and Erb's point must be taken while the shoulder is placed in 90° abduction.

Clinical Application

Ulnar nerve trauma, as well as nerve entrapment in Guyon's canal or behind the medial epicondyle, can be detected using this technique. In addition, the ulnar nerve distal latency is often used in comparison with that of the median nerve in patients with suspected or recovering carpal tunnel syndrome.

Clinical Perspectives

In cases of carpal tunnel syndrome, the distal latency of the median nerve is usually prolonged when compared to equal distance of the ulnar nerve. In polyneuropathy, the distal latency for both the median and the ulnar nerve will be prolonged.

Ulnar (Sensory) Orthodromic Technique Nerve Conduction Study

To determine the nerve conduction velocity of the sensory aspect of the ulnar nerve, the orthodromic technique may be used. In this procedure, the stimulating electrode is applied on the little finger, and the recording electrodes are located at the wrist, elbow, or upper arm.

Electromyograph (EMG) Set-up

Sensitivity/gain: 10–20 μV/div
Filter setting: 100–1000 Hz
Sweep speed: 1 ms/div

Patient Position (Fig. 6–3)

The patient is positioned supine with the arm in 45° abduction.

Recording Electrode Placement (Fig. 6–10)

First recording site (R1):   anterior and most medial aspect of the wrist proximal to the wrist crease close to the flexor carpi ulnaris tendon

Second recording site (R2):   upper one fourth of the medial side of the forearm about 3–4 cm distal to the medial epicondyle

Third recording site (R3):   lower one fourth of the medial side of the arm about 4 cm proximal to the medial epicondyle

Fourth recording site (R4):   medial side of the upper third of the arm between the biceps and triceps muscles

Stimulating Electrode Placement: Standard Technique (Fig. 6–10)

Cathode: MP joint of the little finger
Anode: on distal interphalangeal (DIP) joint of little finger
Ground (green) electrode: on the back of the hand

Stimulating Electrode Placement: Roth Technique (Fig. 6–11)

In this alternative technique the hand-held, two-prong electrical stimulation electrode may be placed between the ring and little fingers at the level of the MP and PIP joints of the closely adducted fingers.

Cathode: proximally placed
Anode: distally placed
Ground (green) electrode: on the back of the hand

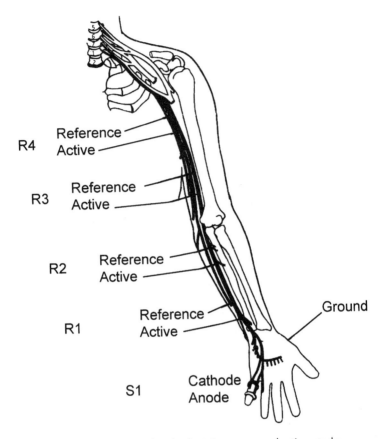

Figure 6–10 Ulnar (sensory) orthodromic nerve conduction study

Electrical Stimulation Parameters

Stimulus duration: 0.1 ms
Stimulus rate: 1 pps
Stimulus intensity: at threshold of maximum sensory action potential

Normal Values

Distal latency: 2.3–3.0 ms
Amplitude: 15–50 μV
Conduction velocity: > 55 meters/second

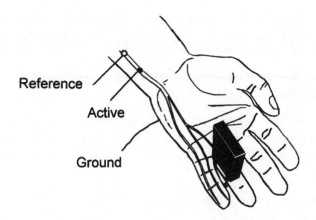

Reference

Active

Ground

Figure 6–11 Roth technique for ulnar (sensory) orthodromic nerve conduction study

Technical Comments

1. Do not allow conducting gel to bridge space between the DIP and PIP of little finger.
2. Average 10 traces while recording the sensory action potential at the wrist level. Recording the sensory nerve potentials at the forearm and arm levels requires averaging more than 10 traces (20–30 traces).
3. Measurement for distance of nerve segment across the elbow must be taken with the elbow in 90° angle.
4. Keep the patient's skin at room temperature (32°C or 90°F) throughout the test.

Clinical Application

Ulnar nerve trauma, as well as nerve entrapment in Guyon's canal or behind the medial epicondyle, can be detected using this technique. In addition, the ulnar nerve distal latency is often used to compare to that of the median nerve in patients with suspected or recovering carpal tunnel syndrome.

Clinical Perspectives

The distal latency of the ulnar nerve would be prolonged when compared to an equally distant segment of the median nerve in cases of ulnar nerve entrapment in Guyon's canal. In polyneuropathy the distal latency for both the median and the ulnar nerve will be prolonged.

Ulnar Nerve (Sensory) Antidromic Technique Nerve Conduction Study

To determine the nerve conduction velocity of the sensory aspect of the ulnar nerve using the antidromic technique, the recording electrodes are taped on the little finger while the stimulating electrodes are located at the wrist, elbow, or upper arm.

Electromyograph (EMG) Set-up

Sensitivity/gain: 10–20 µV/div
Filter setting: 100–1000 Hz
Sweep speed: 1 ms/div

Patient Position

The patient is positioned supine with the arm at 45° in abduction. (See Fig. 6–3.)

Recording Electrode Placement (Fig. 6–12)

Use ring electrodes with conductive gel.

Active (black) electrode: on the MP joint of the little finger
Reference (red) electrode: on the DIP joint of the little finger
Ground (green) electrode: on the back of the hand

Stimulation Sites (Fig. 6–12)

First point (S1):   anteromedial aspect of the wrist proximal to wrist creases and close to the flexor carpi ulnaris tendon
Second point (S2):   anteromedial aspect of the upper one quarter of the forearm and 3–4 cm distal to the medial epicondyle
Third point (S3):   anteromedial aspect of the lower one quarter of the arm and 4 cm proximal to the medial epicondyle
Fourth point (S4):   anteromedial aspect of the upper one quarter of the arm and between the biceps and triceps muscles

Electrical Stimulation Parameters

Stimulus duration: 0.1 ms
Stimulus rate: 1 pps
Stimulus intensity: to elicit maximum sensory action potential

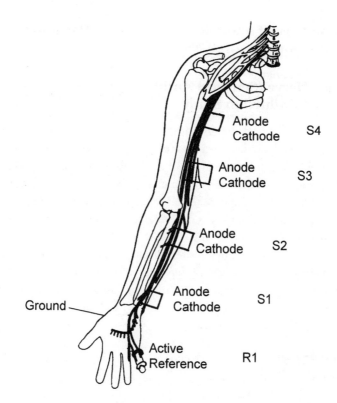

Figure 6–12   Ulnar (sensory) antidromic nerve conduction study

Normal Values

Distal latency: 2.3–3.0 ms
Amplitude: 15–50 μV
Conduction velocity: > 55 meters/second

Technical Comments

1. The sensory conduction velocity should increase in value with more proximal nerve segments due to the increased diameter of the nerve fibers.
2. Keep the patient's skin at room temperature (32°C or 90°F) throughout the testing time.

Clinical Perspectives

The conduction velocity should be comparable when recording by orthodromic or antidromic techniques.

Motor Nerve Conduction Study of the Posterior Interosseous (Radial) Nerve

Anatomic Considerations

The radial nerve is derived from the C5, C6, C7, C8, and T1 spinal nerve roots and the posterior cord of the brachial plexus. The motor branches of the radial nerve motor innervate the triceps brachii, anconeus, brachioradialis, extensor carpi radialis longus, and brevis, as well as the posterior compartment of the forearm (via the posterior interosseous nerve). The sensory branch of the radial nerve arises from the C6–C7 roots and supplies the lateral aspect of the back of the hand. It is most superficial at the lateral humeral epicondyle and at the spiral groove at the middle of the arm.

One of the most common sites for injury to the radial nerve is the lateral epicondyle. Another common site for radial nerve injury is the middle of the humerus following a fracture. The posterior interosseous nerve is commonly entrapped between the two heads of the supinator muscle at the arcade of Frohse.

Electromyograph (EMG) Set-up

Sensitivity/gain: 2–5 mV/div
Filter setting: 10 Hz–2 kHz
Sweep speed: 3 ms/div

Patient Position (Fig. 6–13)

The patient is positioned supine with the arm near the trunk with the hand and forearm rested on the chest.

Recording Electrode Placement (Fig. 6–14)

Active (black) electrode: on motor point of extensor indicis muscle
Reference (red) electrode: dorsal forearm 2 cm distal to active electrode
Ground (green) electrode: dorsal forearm 0.5 cm proximal to active electrode

Ask the patient to perform extension of the index finger and palpate the extensor indicis muscle 3–4 cm proximal to the wrist in the midline between the radius and the ulna.

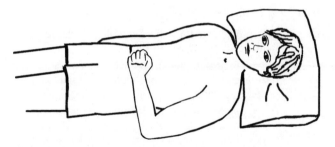

Figure 6–13 Patient position for posterior interosseous branch of the radial nerve conduction study

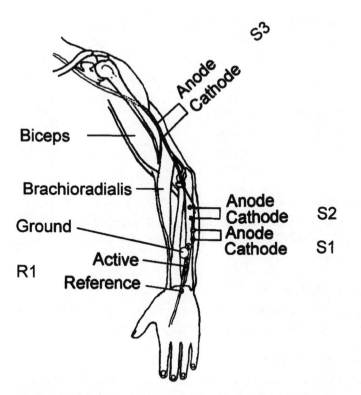

Figure 6–14 Posterior interosseous branch of radial (motor) nerve conduction study

Stimulation Sites (Fig. 6–14)

First point (S1):   5 cm proximal to the active recording electrode on
                      the dorsal surface of the radius

Second point (S2):   10 cm proximal to the first point on the dorsal
                      surface of the radius and about 3 cm distal to the
                      lateral epicondyle

Third point (S3):   10 cm proximal to the second point on the lateral
                      side of the arm between the biceps and triceps
                      muscles and about 4 cm proximal to the lateral
                      epicondyle

Always apply the active (black) stimulation electrode distal to the reference (red) electrode. The hand held, two-prong electrode is easy to use for such a procedure.

Electrical Stimulation Parameters

Stimulus duration: 0.1 ms
Stimulus rate: 1 pps
Stimulus intensity: to elicit maximum motor action potential

Normal Values

Distal latency: 1.5–1.7 ms
Amplitude: 5–7 mV
Conduction velocity: >45 meters/second

Technical Comments

Measurement of the limb segment between the second (below elbow) and third (above elbow) points must be taken while the elbow is at 90° of elbow flexion.

Clinical Applications

The posterior interosseous nerve is frequently entrapped at the arcade of Frohse by radial nerve injuries and by polyneuropathy.

Clinical Perspectives

In patients with entrapment syndrome for the posterior interosseous nerve at the arcade of Frohse, the conduction velocity below the elbow would be significantly lower than that above the elbow.

Radial (Sensory) Nerve Conduction Study

Electromyograph (EMG) Set-up

Sensitivity/gain: 10–20 μV/div
Filter setting: 100–1000 Hz
Sweep speed: 1 ms/div

Patient Position (Fig. 6–13)

The patient is positioned supine with the arm near the trunk and the hand and forearm across patient's chest.

Recording Electrode Placement (Fig. 6–15)

Active (black) electrode: on the dorsal surface of the lower one quarter of the radius, and about 2 cm proximal to the radial styloid process
Reference (red) electrode: 2 cm proximal to the active electrode
Ground (green) electrode: on the dorsal surface of the hand

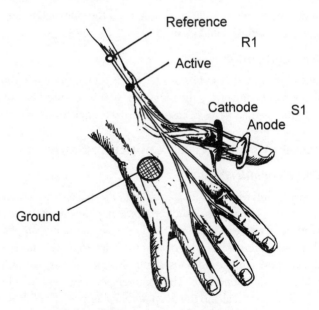

Figure 6–15   Radial (sensory) nerve conduction study

Stimulation Sites (Fig. 6–15)

Use ring stimulating electrodes with conductive gel.

Cathode: MP joint of thumb
Anode: PIP joint of thumb
Ground (green) electrode: dorsum of hand

Stimulation Parameters

Stimulus duration: 0.1 ms
Stimulus rate: 1 pps
Stimulus intensity: to elicit maximum sensory action potential

Average 10 traces for a good representation of radial sensory potential.

Normal Values

Distal latency: 2.0–2.7 ms
Amplitude: 7–15 mV
Conduction velocity: cannot be obtained

Technical Comments

Antidromic recording can be carried out by using the proximally placed electrodes to stimulate while recording from the ring electrodes. (The averaging technique should be used.)

Clinical Application

This technique is used to determine if there is trauma, mononeuropathy, or polyneuropathy involving the radial nerve. It is also used for comparison with the median nerve in cases of carpal tunnel syndrome.

Peroneal (Motor) Nerve Conduction Study

Anatomic Considerations

The peroneal nerves arise from L4, L5 and S1 spinal roots. The common peroneal nerve, sometimes called the lateral popliteal nerve, arises from the sciatic nerve at the popliteal fossa. The sciatic nerve supplies the muscle group of the posterior aspect of the thigh (biceps femoris, semitendinosus, and semimembranosus muscles), as well as partial innervation to the adductor magnus. The common peroneal nerve divides into the superficial peroneal and the deep peroneal nerves after it leaves the popliteal fossa and enters the leg.

The deep peroneal nerve supplies motor innervation to the anterior compartment of the leg that causes dorsiflexion and eversion of the foot (tibialis anterior, extensor digitorum, extensor hallucis longus and brevis, and peroneus tertius muscles). It supplies cutaneous sensation to a small wedge-shaped area between the big toe and the second toe of the dorsum of the foot.

The superficial peroneal nerve supplies motor innervation to the muscles causing eversion and plantar flexion of the foot (peroneus longus and brevis). It supplies cutaneous sensation to the anterolateral aspect of the lower half of the leg and the dorsum of the foot and toes.

The most common sites for injury to the peroneal nerve are at the neck of the fibula, popliteal fossa, or at the anterior aspect of the ankle.

Electromyograph (EMG) Set-up

Sensitivity/gain: 2–5 mV/div
Filter setting: 10 Hz–2 kHz
Sweep speed: 3–5 ms/div

Patient Position (Fig. 6–16)

The patient is positioned supine or side lying with a pillow between the knees.

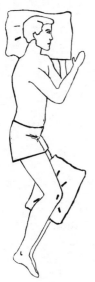

Figure 6–16 Patient position for peroneal and sural nerve conduction studies

Recording Electrode Placement (Fig. 6–17)

Active (black) electrode: on motor point (muscle belly) of extensor digi-
                               torum brevis muscle

Reference (red) electrode: on the MP joint of little toe

Ground (green) electrode: on the dorsum of the foot

To locate the belly of the extensor digitorum brevis on the lateral half
of the dorsum of the foot, ask the patient to perform dorsiflexion of
the toes.

Stimulation Sites (Fig. 6–17)

Apply the active stimulation electrode (cathode) distal to the anode with
2 cm between the two electrodes.

First site (S1):   anterior aspect of lower one quarter of the leg
                       between the tendons for the tibialis anterior and
                       extensor digitorum, and 10 cm proximal to the active
                       electrode

Second site (S2):   behind the neck of the fibula

Third site (S3):   popliteal fossa lateral to midline and 8–10 cm proximal
                    to second site

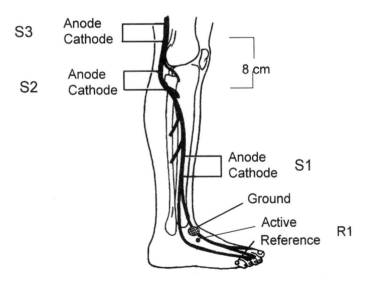

Figure 6–17   Peroneal (motor) nerve conduction study

Stimulation Parameters

Stimulus duration: 0.1 ms
Stimulus rate: 1 pps
Stimulus intensity: to elicit maximum action potential

Normal Values

Distal latency: 3–4.2 ms
Amplitude: 3–7 mV
Conduction velocity: > 40 meters/second

Technical Comments

In the overweight patient, the peroneal nerve is sometimes displaced slightly lateral to the tendons of the tibialis anterior and extensor digitorum muscles. Try to move the stimulator lateral and medial until a maximum response is obtained.

The extensor digitorum brevis (EDB) is sometimes atrophied in women who wear high heels for long periods of their life. In these cases, a small maximum action potential in the EDB may be recorded.

Clinical Applications

This technique is useful in detecting deep peroneal nerve injury at the fibular neck. It is also used to determine the existence of mononeuropathy or polyneuropathy involving the peroneal nerve.

Clinical Perspectives

In cases of deep peroneal nerve compression at the fibular neck, the conduction velocity would be less than normal between the second and third sites with minimal changes between the first and second stimulation sites.

Tibial (Motor) Nerve Conduction Study

Anatomic Considerations

The tibial nerve arises from the L4, L5, and S1, S2 spinal roots and the sciatic nerve at the popliteal fossa. It is the largest division of the sciatic nerve, and it is sometimes called the medial popliteal nerve. It runs in the middle of the popliteal fossa at the back of the knee to supply the muscles of the posterior compartment of the leg that cause plantar flexion of the foot (tibialis posterior, popliteus, flexor digitorum longus and flexor hallucis longus, gastrocnemius, and soleus muscles). The tibial nerve then passes behind and below the medial malleolus where it bifurcates into the medial and lateral plantar nerves. The latter nerves supply the muscles of the plantar surface of the foot.

The common sites for injuries to the tibial nerve are at the popliteal fossa and the medial malleolus where it becomes more superficial.

Electromyograph (EMG) Set-up

Sensitivity/gain: 2–5 mV/div
Filter setting: 10 Hz–2 kHz
Sweep speed: 3–5 ms/div

Patient Position (Fig. 6–18)

Position the patient prone with the lower leg supported in slight flexion with a pillow at the ankle level.

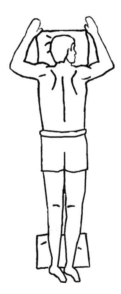

Figure 6–18 Patient position for tibial, medial plantar, and lateral plantar nerve conduction studies

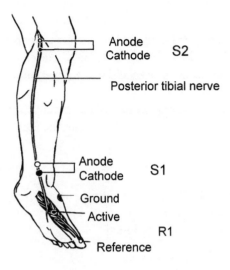

Figure 6-19 Tibial (motor) nerve conduction study

Recording Electrode Placement (Fig. 6-19)

Active (black) electrode: motor point of the flexor hallucis brevis
Reference (red) electrode: MP joint of the hallux
Ground (green) electrode: anterior aspect of the ankle

The active (black) electrode is distal to the reference (red) electrode with at least 2 cm between electrodes.

Stimulation Sites (Fig. 6-19)

First site (S1):   behind the medial malleolus or below it and about 10 cm from the active recording electrode
Second site (S2):   middle of the popliteal fossa

Electrical Stimulation Parameters

Stimulus duration: 0.1 ms
Stimulus rate: 1 pps
Stimulus intensity: to elicit maximum action potential

Normal Values

Distal latency: 4–6 ms
Amplitude: 4–12 mV
Conduction velocity: > 41 meters/second

Technical Comments

The tibial nerve runs in the middle of the popliteal fossa in most patients. In overweight patients, it might be displaced slightly laterally. The clinician needs to move the stimulator laterally or medially until a maximum action potential is obtained.

If a late potential at about 40–45 ms is recorded during stimulation of the tibial nerve at the ankle or knee, it is the H-reflex for the flexor hallucis brevis.

Clinical Applications

This technique is used to determine tibial nerve injury, mononeuropathy, or polyneuropathy. Posterior compartment syndrome or sciatic neuropathy can also be detected using this technique.

Clinical Perspectives

This is the first nerve to show low conduction velocity in patients on dialysis who have a mild degree of neuropathy. The distal latency might be prolonged in patients with tarsal tunnel syndrome with no changes in the conduction velocity.

Lateral Plantar (Motor) Nerve Conduction Study

Anatomical Considerations

The lateral plantar nerve arises from the tibial nerve below the medial malleolus and at the entrance to the foot. It supplies the muscles of the lateral compartment of the sole of the foot (abductor digiti minimi, adductor hallucis, flexor digiti minimi, interossei, quadratus plantae, and the second, third, and fourth lumbrical muscles). It gives sensory cutaneous innervation to the lateral aspect of the sole of the foot and lateral one and half toes. The most common site for injury to the lateral plantar nerve is at the flexor retinaculum.

Electromyograph (EMG) Set-up

Sensitivity/gain: 0.5–1 mV/div
Filter setting   10 Hz–2 kHz
Sweep speed: 3 ms/div

Patient Position (Fig. 6–20a–c)

Position the patient prone with the knee slightly flexed with a pillow at the ankle level or side lying with the tested leg being the upper one.

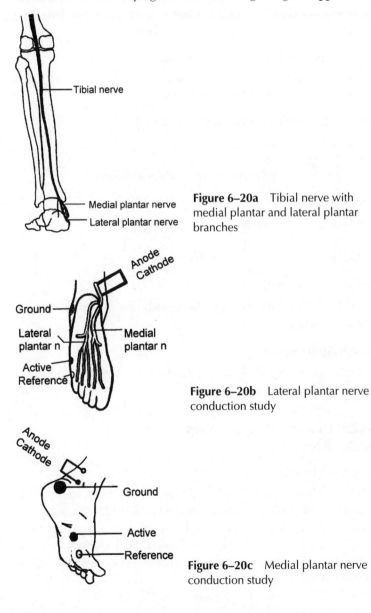

Figure 6–20a Tibial nerve with medial plantar and lateral plantar branches

Figure 6–20b Lateral plantar nerve conduction study

Figure 6–20c Medial plantar nerve conduction study

Recording Electrode Placement (Fig. 6–20b)

Record from the abductor digiti minimi.

Active (black) electrode: 1.5 cm proximal to the MP joint of the little toe
Reference (red) electrode: on lateral side of the MP joint of the little toe
Ground (green) electrode: lateral side of the heel

Stimulation Site (Fig. 6–20b and 6–20c)

First site (S1):   behind the medial malleolus and about 10 cm along the
                   course of the nerve

Electrical Stimulation Parameters

Stimulus duration: 0.1 ms
Stimulation rate: 1 pps
Stimulus intensity: to elicit maximum motor action potential

Normal Values

Distal latency: 4.0 ± 0.5 ms
Amplitude: > 2 mV
Conduction velocity: > 41 meters/second

Technical Comments

The ankle should be at a 90° angle during measurement of the distance of the nerve segment.

Clinical Applications

This technique can be used to detect tarsal tunnel syndrome, mononeuropathy, or tibial nerve injury.

Medial Plantar (Motor) Nerve Conduction Study

Anatomic Considerations

The medial plantar nerve is the distal branch of the tibial nerve below the medial malleolus at the entrance to the sole of the foot. It innervates the muscles of the medial compartment of the foot (flexor digitorum brevis, flexor hallucis brevis, abductor hallucis, and first lumbrical muscles). It also gives cutaneous innervation to the medial side of the plantar surface of the foot.

The most common site of injury to the medial plantar nerve is at the flexor retinaculum, causing tarsal tunnel syndrome.

Electromyograph (EMG) Set-up

Sensitivity/gain: 0.5–1 mV/div
Filter setting: 10 Hz–2 kHz
Sweep speed: 3 ms/div

Patient Position (Fig. 6–18)

Position the patient prone with the knee in slight flexion using a pillow at ankle level or side lying with the tested leg being the lower one.

Recording Electrode Placement (Fig. 6–20c)

Record from the abductor hallucis.

Active (black) electrode: 1 cm below and 1 cm behind the navicular tubercle
Reference (red) electrode: medial side of the MP joint of hallux
Ground (green) electrode: medial side of the heel

Stimulation Site (Fig. 6–20c)

The cathode is distally placed in relationship to the anode.

First site (S1):   behind the medial malleolus and about 8–10 cm along the course of the nerve

Electrical Stimulation Parameters

Stimulus duration: 0.1 ms
Stimulation rate: 1 pps
Stimulus intensity: to elicit maximum motor action potential

Normal Values

Distal latency: 3.7 ± 0.5 ms
Amplitude: > 2 mV
Conduction velocity: > 41 meters/second

Clinical Applications

Tarsal tunnel syndrome, mononeuropathy, or trauma to the tibial nerve can be detected with this technique.

Clinical Perspectives

In tarsal tunnel syndrome, the distal latency would be prolonged, and the amplitude would be smaller than the normal side.

Femoral Nerve Conduction Study

Anatomic Considerations

The femoral nerve originates from L2, L3, and L4 spinal nerve roots. It innervates the iliopsoas, iliacus, pectineus, sartorius, and the quadriceps muscles. It gives cutaneous sensory innervation to the anterior surface of the thigh and medial aspect of the calf. It is most superficial at the inguinal canal at the anterior aspect of the hip.

The most common site for injury to the femoral nerve is at the inguinal canal anterior to the hip joint where it is most superficial.

Electromyograph (EMG) Set-up

Sensitivity/gain: 2–5 mV/div
Filter setting: 10 Hz–2 kHz
Sweep speed: 3–5 ms/div

Patient Position (Fig. 6–21)

The patient is positioned supine with the knee slightly flexed and hip in slight external rotation.

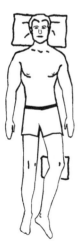

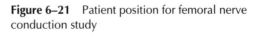

Figure 6–21   Patient position for femoral nerve conduction study

Recording Electrode Placement (Fig. 6–22)

Record from the vastus medialis muscle.

Active (black) electrode:	2 cm proximal and 3 cm medial to the upper border of the patella
Reference (red) electrode:	upper border of the patella
Ground (green) electrode:	anterior surface of the thigh

Stimulation Sites (Fig. 6–22)

The first stimulation site is at the inguinal canal, distal to the inguinal ligament and lateral to the femoral artery. Use a two-prong, hand-held electrode with the active electrode (cathode) distal to the anode. It is sometimes possible to stimulate at a second site above the inguinal ligament.

Stimulation Parameters

Stimulus duration:	0.1 ms
Stimulation rate:	1 pps
Stimulus intensity:	to elicit maximum motor action potential

Normal Values

Distal latency:	3.5–4.5 ms
Amplitude:	5–20 mV
Conduction velocity:	> 45 meters/second

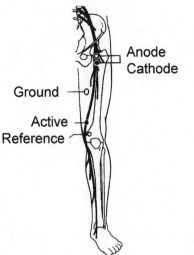

Anode
Cathode
Ground
Active
Reference

Figure 6–22 Femoral (motor) nerve conduction study

Technical Comments

The distal latency may be recorded at the vastus medialis (as presented here) or the rectus femoris muscles. In the latter case, the recording electrodes are placed on the rectus femoris muscle at the front of the thigh, about 14–30 cm from the stimulation electrodes.

Clinical Applications

This technique can be used to determine femoral nerve entrapment at the inguinal level, femoral nerve trauma during hip dislocation, mononeuropathy, or polyneuropathy.

Clinical Perspectives

A compromised femoral nerve may result in a sluggish patellar tendon reflex and buckling of the knee during walking.

Sural (Sensory) Antidromic Nerve Conduction Study

Anatomic Considerations

The sural sensory nerve is formed by the communication between the medial sural cutaneous branch of the tibial nerve and the sural communicating branch of the common peroneal nerve. It runs between the two bellies of the gastrocnemius muscle and distally toward and behind the lateral malleolus to the lateral side of the foot and the little toe. It gives cutaneous sensation to the posterolateral aspect of the leg and the lateral side of the foot. The most common site for injury to the sural nerve is at the lateral aspect of the ankle during sprained lateral ligament with forced foot inversion.

Electromyograph (EMG) Set-up

Sensitivity/gain: 10–20 µV/div
Filter setting: 100–1000 Hz
Sweep speed: 1 ms/div

Patient Position (Fig. 6–16)

The patient is positioned side lying with the tested leg on top of a pillow with the knee and hip flexed.

Recording Electrode Placement (Fig. 6–23)

Active (black) electrode: 1.5 cm distal to the tip of the lateral malleolus
Reference (red) electrode: lateral aspect of the MP joint of the little toe
Ground (green) electrode: on lateral malleolus

Stimulation Site (Fig. 6–23)

First site (S1):   14 cm proximal to the active recording electrode on the
                   course of the nerve at the posterior aspect of the lower
                   one third of the leg

Normal Values

Distal latency: 3.5–4.4 ms
Amplitude: >15 μV

Technical Comments

1. Work the stimulation electrode medially and laterally until the
   maximum action potential is obtained.
2. Orthodromic stimulation of the sural nerve at the lateral side of
   the foot and recording sural sensory potential (in microvolt amplitude) may be overridden by the muscle action potential of the
   soleus muscle (in millivolt amplitude) resulting from the noxious
   stimulation.
3. Average 10 traces for clear action potential.

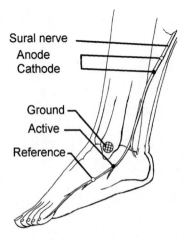

Sural nerve
Anode
Cathode

Ground
Active
Reference

Figure 6–23   Sural (sensory)
antidromic nerve conduction study

Clinical Applications

This technique can be used to detect sural nerve injuries during lateral sprain of the ankle. It is also used to determine mononeuropathy or polyneuropathy involving the sural nerve. The sural nerve is affected early in patients on dialysis with associated neuropathy.

Clinical Perspectives

Compare the symptomatic to the nonsymptomatic leg. The amplitude will decrease and the latency will be prolonged in the symptomatic leg.

References

Sabbahi M, Sedgwick EM: Age-related changes in monosynaptic reflex excitability. *J Gerontol* 37:24–32, 1982.

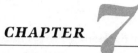

Late Waves

Late wave responses consist of Hoffmann's reflexes (H-reflexes), F waves, and blink reflexes. Late wave responses, so named because of a longer latency than nerve conduction studies, are an important complement to neurophysiologic testing. The late wave responses provide information about the integrity and conduction in the proximal segments of the reflex pathway, such as the plexus and spinal nerve roots.

When a nerve is stimulated, action potentials are generated in the nerve fiber in both directions from the stimulation site. When the action potential travels along the motor axon to the motor neuron with a recurrent discharge in the same cell body, an action potential is generated along the same motor axon back to the innervated muscle fiber. The first motor action potential recorded at the muscle is called the M-response (or M wave). The second action potential, occurring 30–50 ms after stimulation and thus termed a late wave response, is the F wave. The F wave amplitude is small with a latency dependent on the distance between the stimulation site and the spinal cord.

In comparison, if the stimulus activates the sensory axon (1a-afferent), the action potential travels to the spinal cord, where, after a synapse in the ventral horn, some motor neurons are activated. This second-order axon carries the evoked response back to the muscle fibers innervated by that motor neuron. The response recorded at the muscle is called the H-reflex.

H-Reflexes

The H-reflex (also called the Hoffmann response) is considered to be the electrical analog of the tendon reflex (without involvement of the muscle spindle). It can be elicited by electrical stimulation of the Ia afferent fibers while recording the reflex action potential from the muscle supplied by the nerve that has been stimulated. The pathway for the H-reflex (Fig. 7–1) consists of the Ia afferents, alpha motor neurons, and the alpha motor axons to the muscle. This monosynaptic reflex has been used to evaluate the excitability of the alpha motor neurons or the integrity of neural conduction in the afferent–motor neurons–efferent pathway. The H-reflexes can be recorded from the soleus, vastus medialis, flexor hallucis brevis, and flexor carpi radialis muscles. The H-reflex may be used with other procedures, such as tendon vibration or stretching, in order to test neurophysiologic processes pertaining to the excitability of the motor neuron pool such as hypertonia, Parkinson's disease, dystonia, and other central nervous system diseases.

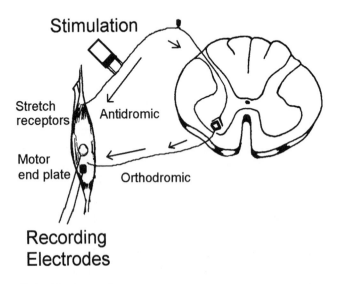

Figure 7–1   H-reflex pathway

During recording of the H-reflex, it is important that the patient is relaxed with an empty bladder and is stress-free, awake, and motionless. The head should remain in the neutral position. When analyzing the H-reflex, clinicians use either the latency or the amplitude to determine the presence of pathologic findings, or sometimes both are used.

Latency

The latency, one of the most important components of the H-reflex, measures the conduction time from the stimulus to the spinal cord synapse, and then to the alpha motor neuron and axon, and extrafusal muscle fibers (Fig. 7–2). The latency is measured from the initial deflection of the electrical stimulation pulse to the initial deflection of the action potential of the H-reflex. For this reason, a longer limb displays a longer latency. Variation in the H-reflex latency between the left and right limb of a patient may be due to a leg length discrepancy or due to comparing the H-reflex latency of each limb when the stimulation sites were not equidistant from the spinal cord. See Figure 7–3, which illustrates the H-reflex normogram (Braddom and Johnson, 1974).

The H-reflex latency does not reflect the degree of compression on the nerve root, but rather significant demyelination, conduction block, or both. The H-reflex latency is prolonged in *chronic* radiculopathy, since impingement of the dorsal root compromises sensory conduction. Proximal neuropathy, Guillain-Barré syndrome, or symptomatic nerve root adhesion with demyelination prolong the central latency of the H-reflex. It is important to note that the H-reflex may appear compromised in the elderly patient, when in fact, the prolonged latency and small amplitude are normal, age-related findings (Sabbahi and Sedgwick, 1982).

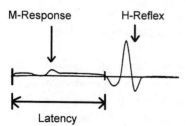

Figure 7–2   Latency of the H-reflex

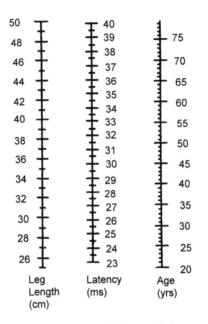

Figure 7–3   H-Reflex normogram (Braddom and Johnson, 1974)

Amplitude

The amplitude of the H-reflex is a reflection of the number of axons activated in the motor efferents by the electrically excited sensory afferents. The current intensity is the amount of current delivered through the stimulation site. The minimal intensity required to allow recording of the H-reflex is called the H-threshold. As the intensity of stimulation is increased, the M-wave response followed by the H-reflex appear on the display screen or oscilloscope. As the intensity is increased, the amplitude of the M wave and H-reflex increase. At one point, the amplitude of the H-reflex no longer increases and is termed the H-maximum. After this point, the H-wave amplitude decreases despite the intensity of stimulation.

    The stimulating electrode must be positioned proximal to the reference anode. This arrangement allows the depolarization signal to travel proximally to the spinal cord without interference from the anode. The recording electrode will detect a lower amplitude of the

H-reflex if inappropriately placed. Similarly, if the stimulation electrode is not accurately located, a painfully high stimulus intensity will be required in order to get the H-maximum.

H-Reflexes of the Lower Extremities

The H-reflexes can be recorded in the lower extremities from the soleus, vastus medialis, and sometimes the flexor hallucis brevis muscles.

The Soleus H-Reflex

The soleus H-reflex, supplied mainly by the S1 spinal segment, can be elicited by electrical stimulation of the tibial nerve at the popliteal fossa. The compound action potentials of the soleus muscle are recorded using surface electrodes. The soleus H-reflex should be tested in both lower extremities using the following procedure.

1. Clean the skin over the calf area and the popliteal fossa behind the knee with alcohol.
2. Use conductive gel for both electrodes. Attach a bar with two surface electrodes about 2 cm distal to the bifurcation of the two heads of the gastrocnemii with the active electrode proximally placed and the reference electrode distally placed. Tape the bar electrode parallel to the longitudinal axis of the leg and in line with the Achilles tendon.
3. Use conductive gel and tape another bar electrode longitudinally in the middle of the popliteal fossa with the active electrode (cathode) proximally placed and the anode distally placed.
4. Use conductive gel and tape a 2.5 cm metal ground electrode over the gastrocnemius between the stimulation and recording sites.
5. Connect the recording electrodes and the ground to the preamplifier and the differential amplifier unit of the electromyograph (EMG) unit (see Fig. 7–5a, for the set-up and electrodes location for the soleus H-reflex).
6. Tell the patient to expect the small electric pulse at the back of the knee to cause involuntary foot plantar flexion. Start the electrical stimulation at a lower amplitude and increase it gradually until plantar flexion of the foot occurs in response to the electrical stimulation. If foot everts, there is erroneous stimulation of the lateral popliteal nerve. In this case, move the stimulation electrode a few millimeters

medially to elicit plantar flexion. Increase the stimulus intensity until
the maximum amplitude of the H-reflex (H-maximum) is reached.
A small M-response will be recorded about 8–10 ms after the stimulus artifact.

7. Ask the patient to refrain from moving his or her head, legs, or
   arms during the test.
8. Using the following procedure, record four representative
   H-maximums in the right lower extremity. Repeat in the left lower
   extremity.

ELECTROMYOGRAPH (EMG) SET-UP

Sensitivity/gain: 1–5 mV/div
Filter setting: 10 Hz–10 kHz
Sweep speed: 5–10 ms/div

PATIENT POSITION (FIG. 7–4):

The patient is prone with the knees slightly flexed by a pillow under the
ankles.

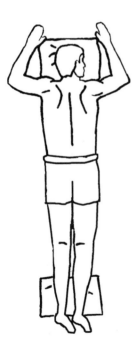

Figure 7–4   Patient position for the soleus
H-reflex

RECORDING ELECTRODE PLACEMENT (FIG. 7–5)

Active (black) electrode: 2 cm distal to the bifurcation of the gastroc-
                             nemii in the midline and in line with
                             Achilles tendon

Reference (red) electrode: Achilles tendon, 2 cm distal to active electrode

Ground (green) electrode: Gastrocnemius

ELECTRICAL STIMULATION SITE (FIG. 7–5)

Cathode: midline of the popliteal fossa

Anode: distally placed using the two-prong electrode

ELECTRICAL STIMULATION PARAMETERS

Stimulus duration: 0.5–1 ms

Stimulus rate: 1 pulse every 5 seconds (0.2 pps)

Stimulus intensity: subthreshold to the action potentials

NORMAL VALUES

Distal latency: 25–32 ms

Peak-to-peak amplitude: 2–12 mV

Shape of action potential: biphasic or triphasic

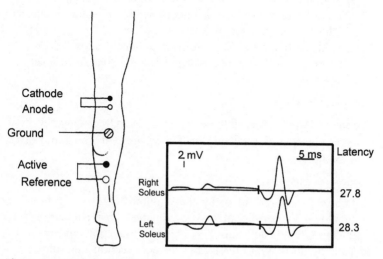

Figure 7–5   Soleus H-reflex

TECHNICAL COMMENTS

1. During stimulation of the tibial nerve, notice the plantar flexion movement of the ankle with contraction of the soleus muscle. If eversion is noted, erroneous stimulation of the peroneal nerve has occurred. Reposition the stimulation electrode medially.

2. Stimulation rates higher than 0.2 pps will cause H-reflex inhibition. Higher intensity will cause H-reflex inhibition with increased muscle action potential.

3. The H-maximum is usually recorded with a minimum M-response that can be recorded at about 8 ms after the stimulus artifact.

4. Test both extremities.

5. Average four H-reflexes for each extremity, and then compare.

6. Patient must be relaxed with legs, arms, and head in one position at all times during the test.

7. Test the H-reflexes from both lower extremities in the standing position and then compare the results to the H-reflexes in the lying position.

8. The distal latency should be within 1.5 ms in both lower extremities.

9. The central latency (from the stimulation site to the spinal cord and back to the stimulation site) can be compared to the distal latency (from the stimulation site to the M-response) by subtraction of the M-response latency from the H-reflex latency.

10. The value for the H-reflex latency depends on the height and age of the patient. (See Figure 7–3.)

11. In older patients, the H-reflex threshold might be as high as the M-response with a more prolonged reflex latency and a smaller amplitude.

CLINICAL APPLICATION

The soleus H-reflex is used to detect lumbosacral radiculopathy, lumbosacral plexopathy, Guillain-Barré syndrome, proximal and distal neuropathies.

CLINICAL PERSPECTIVES

1. In lumbosacral radiculopathy, the amplitude of the soleus muscle should be 50% smaller in the symptomatic limb as compared to the nonsymptomatic limb. This would be more pronounced during standing (loading). In these cases the nerve conduction studies would be normal.

2. Soleus H-reflex suppression was found to be positively correlated with a reduction in the Achilles tendon reflex.
3. The central latency is prolonged in Guillain-Barré syndrome, where the distal latency is prolonged in polyneuropathy. The central latency is prolonged in the symptomatic versus the non-symptomatic limb in patients with lumbosacral radiculopathy.

Vastus Medialis H-Reflex

The vastus medialis H-reflex can be elicited by electrical stimulation of the femoral nerve at the inguinal canal. Stimulation of the femoral nerve, supplied by the L4 spinal segment, causes a compound action potential recorded over the vastus medialis muscle as the H-reflex. Compromise of the L4 root may cause weakness of the quadriceps muscle, reduced patellar tendon reflex, and abnormalities of the vastus medialis H-reflex (Sabbahi and Khalil, 1990).

The protocol to test the vastus medialis H-reflex is as follows.

1. Tape a bar recording electrode with conducting gel in the position described later.
2. Use conductive gel under a ground metal electrode and tape onto the anterior surface of the thigh.
3. Apply the gelled two-prong, hand-held stimulation electrode over the femoral nerve at the inguinal canal.
4. Connect the recording electrodes and the ground electrode to the preamplifier and the differential amplifier of the EMG unit. See the protocol later for the EMG set-up parameters.
5. Inform the patient that he or she will feel an electrical pulse at the inguinal canal with muscle contraction and slight extension of the knee.
6. Start the electrical stimulation with minimal intensity, increasing gradually until there is a mild specific contraction of the vastus medialis muscle. It may be necessary to move the stimulation electrode medially or laterally to elicit a visible muscle contraction. Eliciting the vastus medialis H-reflex requires a stimulus intensity higher than that of the soleus H-reflex because of the depth of the femoral nerve in the inguinal canal.
7. Ask the patient to refrain from movements of the legs, arms, or head during recording.
8. Record four H-reflex maximums from the right lower extremity. Repeat the procedure in the left lower extremity.

ELECTROMYOGRAPH (EMG) SET-UP

Sensitivity/gain: 1–5 mV/div
Filter setting: 10 Hz–10 kHz
Sweep speed: 3–5 ms/div

PATIENT POSITION

Two different testing positions are possible: supine and standing.

RECORDING ELECTRODE PLACEMENT (FIG. 7–6)

Active (black) electrode: belly of the vastus medialis muscle, which is
                                located about 2 cm proximal and 3 cm
                                medial to the upper border of the patella.
                                Position the electrode at a 45° angle to the
                                longitudinal axis of the femur to follow the
                                orientation of the vastus medialis muscle

Reference (red) electrode: upper border of the patella
Ground (green) electrode: front of thigh

ELECTRICAL STIMULATION SITE (FIG. 7–6)

Use the two-prong, hand-held electrode to stimulate the femoral nerve
in the inguinal canal.

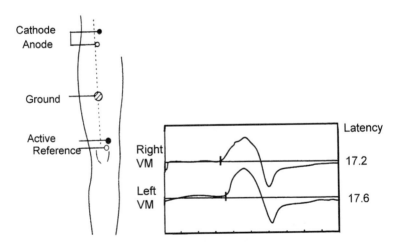

Figure 7–6   Vastus medialis H-reflex

Cathode: proximally in the inguinal canal, distal and medial to the
            inguinal ligament
Anode: distally placed using the two-prong electrode

ELECTRICAL STIMULATION PARAMETERS

Stimulus duration: 0.5–1.0 ms (1 ms is more comfortable)
Stimulus rate: one pulse every 5 seconds (0.2 pps)
Stimulus intensity: at the threshold of muscle (vastus medialis), contrac-
                      tion and mild knee extension

NORMAL VALUES

Distal latency: 15–20 ms
Amplitude: 2–10 mV
Action potential shape: biphasic

TECHNICAL COMMENTS

1. To record the vastus medialis H-reflex in overweight patients a
    higher stimulus intensity may be needed.
2. Stimulation of the femoral nerve is slightly noxious when com-
    pared to the soleus or the FCR H-reflexes.
3. Measure the central latency, and compare to the distal latency.
4. In patients with lumbosacral radiculopathy, compare the H-
    reflexes in supine and standing positions. Standing (spinal loading)
    will be the provocative test for lumbosacral radiculopathy.
5. Test both lower extremities, and compare the amplitude and
    latencies.
6. Average four H-reflexes for each side.
7. Reflex latency in both lower extremities is comparable and
    should be within 1.5 ms of each other.
8. In older patients or those with lumbosacral radiculopathy, the
    threshold of the vastus medialis H-reflexes approaches the
    threshold for the M-response (Sabbahi and Khalil, 1990).
9. Patients must be completely relaxed during testing.
10. The value for the normal latency of the vastus medialis H-reflex
    depends on the height and age of the patient similar to those of
    the soleus H-reflex.

CLINICAL APPLICATIONS

The vastus medialis H-reflex is used to detect lumbosacral radiculopathy due to L4 root compression, femoral nerve entrapment at the
inguinal canal, mononeuropathy and polyneuropathy, Guillain-Barré
syndrome, and proximal neuropathies, or plexopathy.

CLINICAL PERSPECTIVES

1. Suppression of the vastus medialis H-reflex was found to be posi-
    tively correlated to the reduction in the patellar tendon reflex.
2. In lumbosacral radiculopathy due to L4 root compromise, the
    amplitude of the vastus medialis H-reflex in the symptomatic lower
    extremity should be 50% smaller than the nonsymptomatic limb,
    especially during standing (loading). The reflex latency might be
    prolonged, especially in chronic radiculopathy.

Flexor Carpi Radialis H-Reflex (FCR H-Reflex)

The FCR H-reflex is the only H-reflex that can be recorded in the upper
extremity muscles of relaxed normal patients. The FCR muscle is supplied primarily by the C6–C7 spinal roots, which is the cervical spinal segment affected most often with neck pain. The H-reflex can be recorded
in infants or hypertonic hand muscles.

The FCR H-reflex latency reflects the conduction time in the sensory motor pathway of the C6–C7 spinal segment. It may be measured
from the beginning of the stimulus artifact to the deflection (positive or
negative) and measured in milliseconds. The FCR H-reflex latency should
be comparable (within 1 ms) in both upper extremities of the same patient.
Any further discrepancy in the latency between the two upper extremities may indicate abnormalities in the conduction in the more delayed
limb side. On the other hand, between patients the FCR H-reflex latency
may fall within a range of 13–19 ms (Sabbahi and Khalil, 1990).

Prior to electrophysiologic testing, a thorough history must be
obtained to determine the date of onset and the mechanism of injury.
Medical conditions, such as diabetes, metabolic disease, vascular disorders, or neuropathy, should be documented. Diabetic neuropathy may
cause a small amplitude and prolonged latency of the H-reflex. Examination of the deep tendon reflexes and dermatomal sensation should be
performed. Reduction of the triceps brachii tendon reflex has been
directly correlated with a suppression of the FCR H-reflex. The presence
of positive Roo's and Adson's tests would aid in the differential diagnosis
of thoracic outlet syndrome from cervical radiculopathy (Sabbahi and
Jehalil, 1990).

1. Clean the skin of the arm and forearm with alcohol.
2. Attach the ground metal electrode on the lateral side of the upper
    segment of the forearm. Use electroconductive gel and tape.

3. Ask the patient to perform opposition of the thumb and index fingers while flexing the wrist joint. The clinician should give mild resistance to the flexed wrist to locate the FCR muscle on the forearm at about one third of the distance between the medial epidondyle and the radial styloid process.

4. Use the following protocol with a gradual increase in the intensity until an action potential is seen at about 15 ms (the FCR H-reflex). Get the H-maximum by slight increases of the electrical stimulation. A small action potential might be seen at 3 ms (the M-response). Get the H-maximum with the smallest possible M-response.

ELECTROMYOGRAPH (EMG) SET-UP

Sensitivity/gain: 200 µV/div–1 mV/div
Filter setting: 10 Hz–10 kHz
Sweep speed: 3–5 ms/div

PATIENT POSITION (FIG. 7–7)

The patient is positioned supine with the elbow slightly flexed using a pillow under the forearm or, alternatively, the patient is positioned sitting with the elbow flexed to 90° and the supinated forearm supported on the patient's lap.

RECORDING ELECTRODE PLACEMENT (FIG. 7–8)

Attach a bar electrode using conductive gel, and tape to the belly of the FCR muscle.

Active (black) electrode: 3 cm distal and 2 cm lateral to the medial epi-
                            condyle, approximately one fourth of the
                            distance between the medial epicondyle
                            and the radial styloid process
Reference (red) electrode: 2 cm lateral to the active electrode
Ground (green) electrode: on the brachioradialis muscle

ELECTRICAL STIMULATION SITE: (FIG. 7–8)

Cathode: 2 cm proximal and 2 cm lateral to the medial epicondyle (the
           septum between the biceps and brachialis muscles)
Anode: distally placed using the two-prong electrode

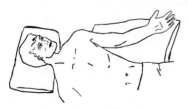

Figure 7–7   Patient position for the flexor carpi radialis (FCR) H-reflex

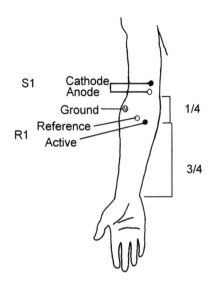

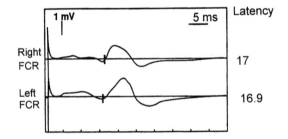

Figure 7–8   Flexor carpi radialis (FCR) H-reflex

ELECTRICAL STIMULATION PARAMETERS

Stimulus duration:	0.5–1.0 ms
Stimulus rate:	pulse every 5 seconds (0.2 pps)
Stimulus intensity:	subthreshold to the action potential (M-response: minimal stimulus intensity)

NORMAL VALUES

Distal latency:	13–19 ms
Amplitude:	0.3–2.5 mV
Action potential shape:	biphasic

TECHNICAL COMMENTS

1. The FCR H-reflex can be recorded in 90% of normal patients.
2. Large variability has been recorded between patients.
3. A small M-response might be recorded at 5 ms in most patients.
4. The difference in stimulus intensity between the H-threshold and H-maximum is very small (a few milliamps).
5. The patient must be completely relaxed during recording.
6. The patient's head should be in the neutral position. Moving the head during testing, will cause an amplitude change of the H-reflex.
7. Average of 4 successful H-reflexes on each limb and compare.
8. Test the patient during lying (unloading) and sitting (loading) and compare, especially in patients with cervical radiculopathy.
9. Measure the central latency (H/latency − M/latency) and compare to distal latency (M/latency). It should be prolonged in the symptomatic limb.
10. Reflex latencies in both lower extremities are comparable and should be within 1ms in normal patients.
11. The normal value for the FCR H-reflex latency depends on the length of the upper limb and the age of the subjects.

CLINICAL APPLICATIONS

The FCR H-reflex may be used to detect cervical radiculopathy, mononeuropathy and polyneuropathy, plexopathy, spinal root avulsion, or injuries.

CLINICAL PERSPECTIVES

1. In cervical radiculopathy, the H-reflex amplitude of the symptomatic limb should be 50% smaller than the amplitude of the nonsymptomatic limb. In chronic conditions, the reflex latency would be prolonged in the symptomatic versus nonsymptomatic conditions (Sabbahi and Khalil, 1990)
2. In proximal neuropathies the central latency would show slower conduction when compared to the distal latency.

Kinesiologic H-Reflex for the Evaluation and Treatment of Radiculopathy

Postural modifications, leading to compression or decompression of the spinal root, can be objectively determined using the H-reflex. Studies have demonstrated the effect of neck position on the foramen of the vertebrae. For example, forward bend (flexion) of the neck increases the foraminal dimension, whereas backward bend (extension) decreases the foraminal dimension. Side bend (lateral bend) has been postulated to close the intervertebral foraminae on the concave side and increase the foraminal dimension on the convex side of the bend (Krag, 1997). Retraction, traction, or gentle oscillated rotation with neck extension have all successfully reduced radicular symptoms in the clinic.

In patients with L4 radiculopathy, the amplitude of the H-reflex on the symptomatic limb is significantly reduced over that of the contralateral limb during standing. These observations led to the hypothesis that unloading the spine in the lying (supine) position would provide a mechanical and gravitational advantage over the position of sitting or standing in terms of nerve decompression. Using the FCR H-reflex as an objective measure of compression, it was found that bilateral relative suppression of the H-reflex occurs during loading of the normal spine in the sitting position.

In patients with cervical radiculopathy, there is more reflex suppression in the symptomatic limb than the contralateral side with the degree of reflex suppression directly related to the degree of compromise within the spinal root (Sabbahi and Khalil, 1990; Sabbahi and Abdulwahab, 1999). The H-reflex, recorded at the FCR, is useful in differentiating C7 radiculopathy from thoracic outlet syndrome or carpal tunnel syndrome. This reflex, however, is present in only 90% of the population, such that the absence of the FCR H-reflex in nonsymptomatic patients is not considered a pathologic finding.

The peak-to-peak amplitude of the H-reflex is initially affected in lumbosacral or cervical radiculopathy with the amplitude of the symptomatic limb 50% smaller than that of the nonsymptomatic limb. Compromised conduction of the H-reflex signal through the impingement site of the symptomatic side results in a reduction of the peak-to-peak amplitude, directly related to the degree of axonal damage or loss (Fig. 7–9). The amplitude of the H-reflex is so sensitive to compression of the nerve that simple postural changes immediately affect this parameter. In the lying position, body weight and the gravitational forces on the spinal nerve roots are diminished with a resultant decrease in radicular symptoms (Fig. 7–10). It is, therefore, necessary to test the H-reflex in a provocative position, such as in sitting or standing, once the H-reflex in the lying (supine) position has been attained (Fig. 7–11).

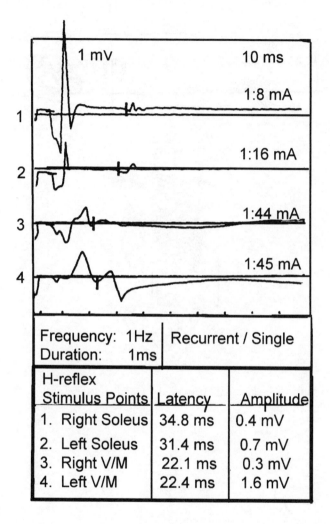

Figure 7–9   Soleus and vastus medialis H-reflex of right and left legs

Testing the kinesiologic H-reflex in different postures will determine the optimum spinal posture (OSP). The OSP is the position that allows maximum decompression of the spinal nerve root whereas the unwanted spinal posture (USP) describes the position that may cause further compression of the affected spinal nerve root. Avoidance of the USP and promotion of the OSP in exercises, as well as activities

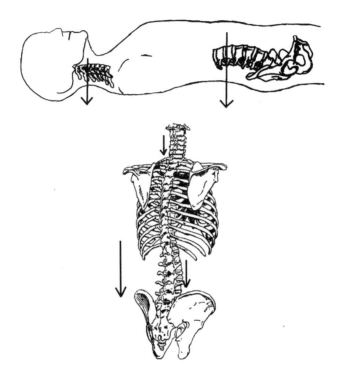

Figure 7–10   Gravitational forces on the spinal nerve roots in supine position

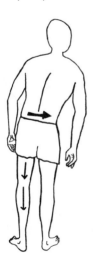

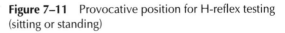

Figure 7–11   Provocative position for H-reflex testing (sitting or standing)

of daily living, reduces neural irritation, edema, and radicular symptoms and promotes recovery of the compromised nerve root. For example, patients with an OSP of right sidebend must sleep on a soft mattress on their left side to cause vertebral column curvature toward the right side. The OSP depends on the pathology, duration of occurrence, spinal level affected, and the degree of spinal nerve root compression. In the lower extremity, 50% of the patients may demonstrate an OSP of a single plane of movement (i.e, around a single axis). In the other half of the population, an increase in the H-reflex amplitude may be reflected by a combination of movements, one of which includes rotation (referred to as a double axes OSP). In the OSP, there should be a reduction in the patient's report of pain and radicular symptoms with an observable increase in the amplitude of the H-reflex; therefore, do not force the patient to move into or through the painful range (Abdulwahab and Sabbahi, 1999).

In addition, the kinesiologic H-reflex may identify other spinal postures that cause relative degrees of reflex recovery (favored posture) or reflex suppression (unfavored posture). These findings should be incorporated in the treatment exercises and in positional recommendations for the patient.

Periodic testing of the H-reflex is important to monitor remyelination of the compromised nerve root. If the correct OSP is not adopted during this period, it will be evident during periodic H-reflex testing and can be dealt with accordingly. It takes several weeks after elimination of radicular symptoms before complete remyelination of the spinal root occurs. Thus, it is important for the patient to continue the positional and exercise program. Remyelination is complete when there is an increase in the H-reflex amplitude in the neutral position. The patient must continue the daily OSP exercises for 1 month. After complete elimination of the radicular symptoms, a general endurance and strengthening program, such as walking 30 minutes a day, is recommended.

Kinesiologic H-Reflex to Determine Optimum Spinal Posture (OSP)

Using a repetitive automatic electrical stimulation at 0.2–0.5 pps, the kinesiologic H-reflex is measured during postural changes of the head or trunk and includes loading or unloading of the spine. The findings from this test aid in the determination of the optimum spinal posture (OSP), the unwanted spinal posture (USP), the favored posture (FP), and the unfavored posture (UP). In the completely relaxed patient, the neck or trunk is passively moved to the end-range of double or single-axis motions and held in this position for 10 seconds prior to H-reflex recording.

Cervical (FCR) Kinesiologic H-Reflex

1. Test the FCR H-reflex in the right, then the left arms in the lying (supine) position with neutral head position. Record the H-maximum, and store it on the screen.
2. Keep the stimulation and recording electrodes in place while moving the patient to the sitting position. Test the H-reflex in the neutral head position from the right and then the left side. Record the maximum FCR H-reflex in this spinal-loaded position, and store it on the screen. Make sure that the amplitude of the M-response is the same as during the lying position. Normally there is a relative reduction in the peak-to-peak amplitude of the H-reflex during sitting as compared to the amplitude recorded in the lying position. In the case of a compromised nerve root, there would be more reflex suppression on the symptomatic side.
3. With the patient in the sitting position, passively move the patient's head within a pain-free range to the end-feel of side bend to the right. Hold for 10 seconds. Record four reflexes, and compare them to the stored FCR H-reflex.
4. Repeat step 3 for side bend to the left.
5. Repeat step 3 for forward bend (flexion).
6. Repeat step 3 for backward bend (extension).
7. Repeat step 3 for rotation to the right side.
8. Repeat step 3 for rotation to the left side.
9. Repeat step 3 for neck retraction.
10. Repeat step 3 for neck protraction.
11. Repeat step 3 for right side bend followed by rotation to the right side.
12. Repeat step 3 for right side bend followed by rotation to the left side.
13. Repeat step 3 for left side bend followed by rotation to the right side.

14. Repeat step 3 for left side bend followed by rotation to the left side.
15. Repeat step 3 for forward and backward bend followed by rotation to the right and left side.

Note: The FCR H-reflex amplitude varies between 0.5–2.5 mV (Sabbahi and Khalil, 1990). In normal patients, forward bend of the neck caused H-reflex suppression, whereas backward bend, side bend, or rotation toward the side of the recording electrodes produced higher reflex facilitation (Sabbahi and Abdulwahab, 1999).

Lumbosacral Kinesiologic H-Reflex

The soleus (S1) or vastus medialis (L4) kinesiologic H-reflex can be determined using the following positions.

1. Test the soleus (or vastus medialis) H-reflex in the right leg, then the left leg in the lying position with a neutral spine position. Record the H-maximum, and store it on the screen.
2. Keep the stimulation and recording electrodes in place while moving the patient to the standing position. The patient must distribute his or her weight equally on both legs and look straight ahead without moving during reflex recording. Test the H-reflex from the right, then the left side. Record the maximum soleus (or vastus medialis) H-reflex in this spinal-loaded position. Make sure that the amplitude of the M-response is the same as during the lying position. The H-reflex in the standing position is normally suppressed as compared to the lying position. The reflex suppression should be symmetric in both lower extremities if pathology-free (Ali and Sabbahi, 2000). Patients with radiculopathy demonstrate asymmetric H-reflexes with the symptomatic leg displaying a suppressed kinesiologic H-reflex over that of the nonaffected leg.
3. With the patient in the standing position, passively move the patient's trunk within a pain-free range to the end-feel of side bend to the right. Hold for 10 seconds. Record four reflexes, and compare them to the stored H-reflex on the screen.
4. Repeat step 3 for side bend to the left.
5. Repeat step 3 for forward bend (flexion).
6. Repeat step 3 for backward bend (extension).
7. Repeat step 3 for rotation to the right side.

8. Repeat step 3 for rotation to the left side.
9. Repeat step 3 for right side bend followed by rotation to the right side.
10. Repeat step 3 for right side bend followed by rotation to the left side.
11. Repeat step 3 for left side bend followed by rotation to the right side.
12. Repeat step 3 for left side bend followed by rotation to the left side.
13. Repeat step 3 for forward and backward bend followed by rotation to the right and left side.

For any of the kinesiologic H-reflexes the following procedure can be used.

1. Identify the position that causes the maximum recovery of the compromised H-reflex and call this the OSP. Patients should be encouraged to adopt this posture for exercise and activities of daily living.
2. Identify the position(s) that cause further H-reflex suppression, and call these the unwanted spinal posture(s) (USP). Patients should be discouraged from exercises or moving toward such posture(s).
3. Identify the positions that cause a relative suppression of the H-reflex, and call these unfavored postures (UP). Those positions that cause a slight recovery of the H-reflex are called favored postures (FP).

Ask the patient to report the intensity of his or her radicular symptoms using an analog scale. Then the patient should maintain the end-range of the OSP for 10 minutes and report the intensity of the radicular symptoms again. The patient should be instructed to perform repeated oscillatory exercises at the end-range of the OSP for 10 minutes immediately before going to bed and immediately upon waking in the morning, in addition to three more times during the day. In addition, patients should sleep in the OSP for 30 minutes and adopt the OSP for activities of daily living or prolonged sitting or standing postures.

F Waves

The F wave is elicited by stimulation of the muscle's nerve supramaximally so that the alpha axons are stimulated. The signal travels antidromically to excite the alpha motor neurons. A response is sent back along the same alpha motor neuron to the muscle, causing a contraction. Therefore, the pathway for the F wave is back and forth along the same alpha motor axons (Fig. 7–12). The F wave, which can be recorded from almost all superficial skeletal muscles, has a small amplitude compared with the M-response or the H-reflex (Fisher, 1992).

Clinical Applications

The F wave can be used to detect thoracic outlet syndrome, carpal tunnel syndrome, motor neuropathy, proximal neuropathy, plexopathy, Guillain-Barre syndrome, amyotrophic lateral sclerosis, stroke, peripheral nerve injury, pelvic/shoulder girdle tumors, space occupying lesions, nerve root avulsion, or postoperative nerve root adhesion. In thoracic outlet syndrome, the F wave for the ulnar nerve innervating the abductor digiti minimi (ADM) is prolonged when compared to that of the median nerve innervating the abductor pollicis brevis (APB) for equal nerve segments. In carpal tunnel syndrome, the F wave for the APB (median nerve) is prolonged when compared to the ADM (ulnar nerve) F wave. The ulnar nerve F wave (ADM) will be delayed in patients with

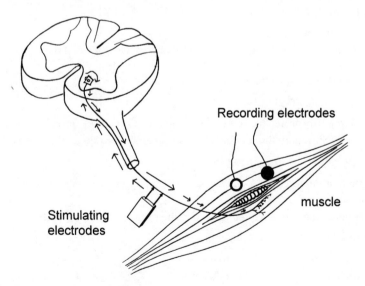

Figure 7–12   F-wave pathway

Guillain-Barré syndrome and proximal neuropathy. The F wave in stroke patients will display an increased amplitude due to increased motor neuron excitability.

Patients with adhered nerve roots after spinal surgery will display a dramatically delayed F wave. In motor neuropathy, the F-wave latency would be prolonged more than the H-reflexes. In plexopathy, the latency of the flexor hallucis brevis F wave is markedly increased with changes in the proximal conduction velocity.

F Waves of the Upper Extremities

F Waves of the Abductor Pollicis Brevis (Median Nerve)

ELECTROMYOGRAPH (EMG) SET-UP

Sensitivity/gain: 200–500 µV/div
Filter setting: 10 Hz–10 kHz
Sweep speed: 5 ms/div

PATIENT POSITION

The patient is positioned supine with the arm in 45° abduction.

RECORDING ELECTRODE PLACEMENT

Active (black) electrode: belly of the APB
Reference (red) electrode: metacarpal phalangeal (MP) joint of the thumb
Ground (green) electrode: back of the hand

ELECTRICAL STIMULATION SITE

Use the two-prong, handheld electrode with the cathode proximal to the anode. Stimulate the median nerve at the anterior aspect of the wrist.

ELECTRICAL STIMULATION PARAMETERS

Stimulus duration: 0.1–0.5 ms
Stimulus rate: 1 pps
Stimulus intensity: suprathreshold to the muscle action potential

NORMAL VALUES (FIG. 7–13)

Distal latency: < 30 ms
Amplitude: 0.2–0.5 mV
Action potential shape: biphasic or multiphasic

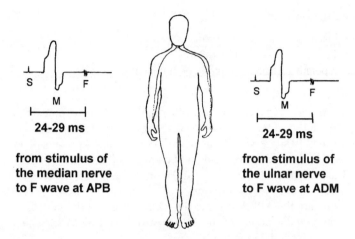

Figure 7–13   F-wave normal values for the abductor pollicis brevis (APB) and the abductor digiti minimi (ADM)

F Waves of the Abductor Digiti Minimi (Ulnar Nerve)

ELECTROMYOGRAPH (EMG) SET-UP

Sensitivity/gain: 200–500 µV/div
Filter setting: 10 Hz–10 kHz
Sweep speed: 5 ms/div

PATIENT POSITION

The patient is positioned supine with the arm in 45° abduction.

RECORDING ELECTRODE PLACEMENT

Active (black) electrode: belly of the ADM
Reference (red) electrode: MP joint of the little finger
Ground (green) electrode: back of the hand

ELECTRICAL STIMULATION SITE

Use the two-prong, handheld electrode with the cathode proximal to the anode. Stimulate the ulnar nerve at the anteromedial side of the wrist.

ELECTRICAL STIMULATION PARAMETERS

Stimulus duration: 0.1–0.5 ms
Stimulus rate: 1 pps
Stimulus intensity: suprathreshold to the muscle action potential

NORMAL VALUES (FIG. 7–13)

Distal latency: < 31 ms
Amplitude: 0.2–0.5 mV
Action potential shape: biphasic or multiphasic

TECHNICAL COMMENTS

1. If experiencing difficulty recording the ulnar F wave, quickly stretch the ADM before delivering the electrical stimulation.
2. Record 10 successful F waves, and measure the shortest latency.
3. Test both upper extremities, and compare.
4. Calculate the central latency and motor conduction velocity, and compare for both extremities.
5. Compare the APB F wave to the ADM F wave of the same limb.
6. Compare the latency of the APB F wave for equal distance nerve segments on the same limb.
7. The amplitude of the F wave has relatively less clinical meaning.

F Waves of the Lower Extremities

The F waves are commonly recorded in the lower extremity from the extensor digitorum brevis (EDB) (peroneal nerve) and from the flexor hallucis brevis (tibial nerve).

F Wave for the Extensor Digitorum Brevis (EDB) (Peroneal Nerve)

ELECTROMYOGRAPHY (EMG) SET-UP

Sensitivity/gain: 200–500 µV/div
Filter setting: 10 Hz–10 kHz
Sweep speed: 10 ms/div

PATIENT POSITION

The patient is positioned supine.

RECORDING ELECTRODE PLACEMENT (FIG. 7–14)

Active (black) electrode: belly of extensor digitorum brevis
Reference (red) electrode: lateral aspect of the MP joint of little toe
Ground (green) electrode: dorsum of foot

ELECTRICAL STIMULATION SITE

Using the two-prong, handheld electrode with the cathode proximal to the reference electrode, stimulate the peroneal nerve at the front of the ankle using the following protocol.

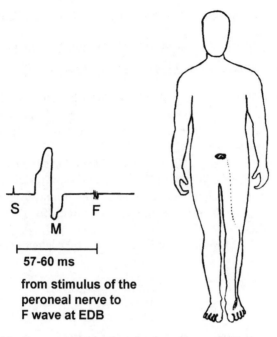

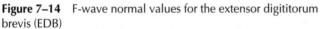

S   **F**

M

57-60 ms

**from stimulus of the
peroneal nerve to
F wave at EDB**

Figure 7–14   F-wave normal values for the extensor digititorum
brevis (EDB)

ELECTRICAL STIMULATION PARAMETERS

Stimulus duration: 0.1–0.5 ms
Stimulus rate: 1.0 pps
Stimulus intensity: suprathreshold to the action potential (M-response)

NORMAL VALUES

Distal latency: < 56 ms
Amplitude: 0.2–1.0 mV
Action potential shape: biphasic or multiphasic

TECHNICAL COMMENTS

1. If difficulty occurs attempting to elicit the F wave for the EDB
   muscle, stretch the three lateral toes before giving the electrical
   stimulus.
2. Test both lower extremities.
3. Record 10 consecutive F waves for each limb. Measure and record
   the latency to the deflection of the earliest F-wave response.

4. The F wave has a variable latency within 2.0 ms for 10 consecutive traces.
5. Compare the F-wave latency for the EDB to those of the flexor hallucis brevis (FHB) on the same limb using equal distance nerve segments.
6. The amplitude of the F wave has relatively less clinical value.
7. To calculate the conduction time from the stimulation site to the spinal cord (only half of the pathway) divide the value for the central latency by two.
8. Measure the distance (in millimeters) from the stimulation site to the vertebral column at L5. Since the F wave travels along the motor axons antidromically and then orthodromically, the measured distance should be doubled when calculating the conduction velocity.
9. Subtract the M-response latency from the total latency of the F wave minus one.

$$\frac{D \times 2\,(mm)}{F - M - 1\,(ms)}$$

F Waves of the Flexor Hallucis Brevis (FHB) (Tibial Nerve)

ELECTROMYOGRAPH (EMG) SET-UP

Sensitivity/gain: 200–500 µV/div
Filter setting: 10 Hz–10 kHz
Sweep speed: 10 ms/div

PATIENT POSITION

The patient is positioned supine.

ELECTRODE PLACEMENT (FIG. 7–15)

Active (black) electrode: 2 cm proximal to the MP joint of the hallux and on the belly of the flexor hallucis brevis
Reference (red) electrode: MP joint of the hallux
Ground (green) electrode: dorsum of foot

ELECTRICAL STIMULATION

Electrical stimulation of the tibial nerve behind the medial malleolus. Use the two-prong, handheld electrode with the active cathode proximal to the reference anode.

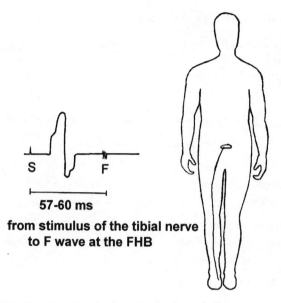

S   F

57-60 ms
from stimulus of the tibial nerve
to F wave at the FHB

Figure 7–15   F-wave normal values for the flexor hallucis
brevis (FHB)

ELECTRICAL STIMULATION PARAMETERS

Stimulus duration: 0.1–0.5 ms
Stimulus rate: 1 pps
Stimulus intensity: supramaximal to the action potential (M-response)

NORMAL VALUES (FIG. 7–15)

Distal latency: < 60 ms
Amplitude: 0.5–1 mV
Action potential shape: multiphasic

Blink Reflex

The blink reflex is a commonly used brain stem reflex involving contraction of the orbicularis occuli following electrical stimulation of the supraorbital nerve at the medial side of the upper margin of the orbital cavity. The afferent limb of the blink reflex pathway is cranial nerve V (trigeminal nerve). The efferent pathway is cranial nerve VII (facial nerve).

ELECTROMYOGRAPH (EMG) SET-UP

Sensitivity/gain: 200–500 μV/div
Filter setting: 10 Hz–10 kHz
Sweep speed: 5 ms/div

PATIENT POSITION

The patient is positioned supine or sitting with the head resting.

RECORDING ELECTRODE PLACEMENT (FIG. 7–16A)

Active electrode (black):   lateral corner of the orbital cavity
Reference electrode (red):   lateral side of the nasal bone
Ground (green):   front and lateral side of the forehead

The recording can be carried out from the ipsilateral side of the stimulation (single channel recording), as well as from the contralateral side (two channel recording).

ELECTRICAL STIMULATION (FIG. 7–16A)

Stimulation of the supraorbital nerve at the anteromedial side of the upper margin of the orbital cavity with the cathode on the nerve and the anode located 2 cm superior to the active electrode on the forehead. Use the two-prong, hand-held electrode for convenience of stimulation.

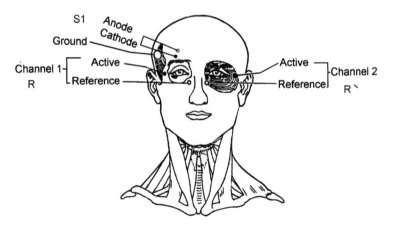

Figure 7–16a   Blink reflex electrode placement

ELECTRICAL STIMULATION PARAMETERS

Stimulus duration: 0.1 ms
Stimulus rate: one pulse every 5 seconds (0.2 pps)
Stimulus intensity: small amplitude intensity at threshold of eye blinking

NORMAL VALUES (FIG. 7–16B)

Latency to R1:   9–11 ms
Latency to R2:   29–35 ms
Amplitude (R1 and R2):   not useful clinically
Action potential shape (R1):   biphasic or triphasic
Action potential shape (R2):   multiphasic that lasts for more than 10 ms

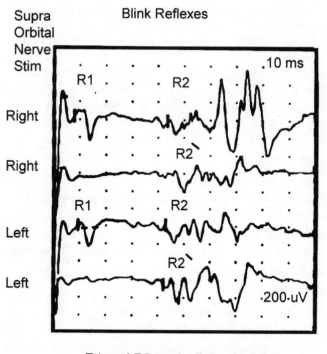

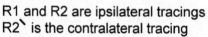
R1 and R2 are ipsilateral tracings
R2` is the contralateral tracing

Figure 7–16b   Blink reflex measurements

Electrical stimulation of the right supraorbital nerve results in recording R1 and R2 on the ipsilateral side (upper trace Fig. 7-16b). Stimulation of the left supraorbital nerve results in recording R2′ on the contralateral side (sound trace, right side, Fig. 7-16b). Similar recordings are made from the left orbicularis occuli muscles while stimulation is applied ipsilaterally (third trace, Fig. 7-16b) and contralaterally (fourth trace, Fig. 7-16b). The first response, called the R1 response, represents the time of conduction along the trigeminal and facial nerve, and is always absent on the contralateral side. The second response, R2, represents the time of conduction along the trigeminal pontine relay and facial nerve. R2′ can be recorded by stimulation of the contralateral supraorbital nerve. It represents the signal crossing to the contralateral side of the brain stem.

TECHNICAL COMMENTS

1. The blink reflex is subject to accommodation; therefore, it is important to obtain the reflex within the first five stimuli.
2. Compare the reflex latency of the ipsilateral to the contralateral recordings.
3. R2 latency is highly variable. Use the shortest latency value.
4. The latency of the R2 potential is variable and the duration and amplitude may vary due to changing excitability of the motor-neuron pool. Thus, some clinicians average the amplitude of both the ipsilateral and contralateral sides.

CLINICAL APPLICATIONS

The blink reflex is useful in measuring the level of consciousness and depth of anesthesia in the operating room. It is also used to assist in the differential diagnosis of brain stem pathologies, Bell's palsy and other facial nerve injuries, trigeminal neuralgia, acoustic neuroma, Guillain-Barré syndrome, multiple sclerosis, Charcot-Marie-Tooth disease, and whiplash injuries with dizziness.

CLINICAL PERSPECTIVES

Patients with brain stem contusions after whiplash injury present with a prolonged latency of R2 on the ipsilateral, as well as the contralateral side of the stimulation. In patients with Bell's palsy, the amplitude of R2 is decreased or the R2 may be delayed. In patients with a tumor on the right brain stem, R1 and R2 for ipsilateral stimulation on the left side would be normal, but R2 for ipsilateral stimulation of the right side would be prolonged. In addition, R2 for contralateral stimulation on both sides would be prolonged due to the delayed transmission through the tumor site.

References

Ali A and Sabbahi M: H reflex changes under spinal loading and unloading conditions in cervical subjects. *Clin Neurophysiology* 111:1–7, 2000.

Braddom RI, Johnson EW: Standardization of H-reflex and diagnostic use in S-1 radiculopathy. *Arch Phys Med Rehabil* 55:161–166, 1974.

Fisher M: H-reflexes and F-waves: Physiology and clinical indications. AAEM #13. *Muscle and Nerve* 15:1223, 1992.

Krag M: Biomechanics of the cervical spine: 1 General Trauma. In J Frymeyer, ed. *The Adult Spine: Principles and Practice.* New York: Lippincott-Raven, 1997, p. 1075.

Sabbahi M, Abdulwahab S: Cervical root compression monitoring by flexor carpi radialis. *Spine* 24:137–141, 1999.

Sabbahi M, Khalil M: Segmental H-reflex studies in upper and lower limbs in patients with radiculopathy. *Arch Phys Med Rehabil* 71:223–227, 1990.

Sabbahi M, Sedgwick EM: Age-related changes in monosynaptic reflex excitability. *J Gerontol* 37:24–32, 1982.

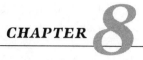

Electrical Stimulation of Denervated Muscles

Electrical stimulation of denervated muscle has been used for over a century in an effort to keep the muscle viable, limit edema, and delay muscle fibrosis while the nerve regenerates. Denervation results in biochemical and trophic changes that affect the contractile properties of the muscle (Spielholz, 1991). Biochemical changes occur in the sarcoplasm and sarcoplasmic reticulum that decrease the resting potential from -80 mV to -65 mV (Albuquerque and McIsaac, 1970; Guth et al, 1981). The neuromuscular junction begins to degenerate, causing a prolonged chronaxie in the strength–duration curve, an increase in contraction time, and a decrease in the tension of the contraction. This may be due, in part, to increased sensitivity to acetylcholine at the neuromuscular junction as well as the entire length of the fiber's membrane (Axelsson and Thesleff, 1959).

During the period of denervation, the muscle fibers atrophy at a species-specific rate that can be correlated with the metabolic rate and life span of the mammal (Cummins, 1992). Skeletal muscle undergoes a 30–60% loss in weight in the first month after denervation (Gutmann and Zelena, 1962; Sunderland, 1978); however, the rate of muscle atrophy is higher if the species has a high metabolic rate and short life expectancy (Knowlton and Hines, 1936). In animals, atrophy can be measured by microscopic analysis of the fiber or by dissection and weight of the isolated muscle. Weighing the muscle does not account for compensatory factors, such as hypertrophy of the remaining fibers, or the weight of fibrous tissue and edema as a result of the injury. The research findings of denervated muscle in the laboratory animal are difficult to compare with the effect of denervation in human muscle.

In the human, if the muscle fibers are not reinnervated within 3 years, the contractile elements of the muscle will be replaced by fibrous connective tissue (Bowden and Gutmann, 1944; Cummings, 1992). Reattachment of an amputated part, requiring microsurgery to repair severed vascular, neurologic, and bony components, is only the beginning of the healing process. Following reattachment, the muscles remain paralyzed for months or years until the nerves regenerate and reinnervate the muscle. If the tissues and bones heal but the muscle remains denervated, volitional motor control of the affected muscle will not return (Spielholz, 1991).

Denervated muscle appears to have some plasticity in response to electrical stimulation for a *short* interval prior to reinnervation. During this period, low frequency electrical stimulation applied to rabbit muscle has been shown to prevent atrophy and increase resistance to fatigue for a short period of time (Girlanda et al, 1982; Nix, 1982; Nix et al, 1985). Ironically, electrical stimulation for more than 6 weeks will *increase* the rate of atrophy of type I fibers (Girlanda et al, 1982; Gutmann and Gutmann, 1944).

If reinnervation is expected within 1 year or 18 months in the human patient, electrotherapy to prevent muscle degeneration is not necessary. In fact, it may be detrimental to reinnervation, as is the case with electrical stimulation to a transplanted muscle (Jansen et al, 1973). In addition, electrical stimulation is not recommended for partial lesions because terminal axonal sprouting will be impeded (Brown and Holland, 1979; Herbison et al, 1973; Pachter et al, 1982; Schimrigk et al, 1977). Thus, it is the current philosophy that for transplanted muscles or partial denervation it is more important to limit edema and stasis, maintain flexibility, and avoid further injury to the muscles (Speilholz, 1991).

Many studies have been performed to determine the optimal conditions for electrical stimulation of completely denervated muscle. The effects depend on the current, pulse duration, waveform, frequency, amplitude, placement of the electrodes, position of the muscle at the initiation of stimulation (stretched, resting length, or shortened), onset of electrical stimulation from the time of denervation, number of contractions obtained during stimulation, amplitude in terms of producing a visible muscle contraction versus joint movement, contraction against resistance, type of muscle contraction (twitch versus tetanus), length of rest between contractions, number of sessions per day, total number of sessions provided, and length of time electrotherapy was provided after denervation (days, months, years). There is a paucity of well-controlled research studies on electrical stimulation of human denervated muscle; and, thus, controversy continues to exist on the best parameters for its use in a clinical setting.

It is generally accepted that a monophasic current is more beneficial than a biphasic current if all other parameters remain unchanged. Low frequency electrical stimulation (10–30 pps) is commonly used. The pulse duration has been reported to be the most critical parameter for electrical stimulation of completely denervated muscle. If the chronaxy of the muscle is known from a recent strength–duration curve, that value should be used for the pulse duration (Cummins, 1992). If the chronaxy is not known, however, the pulse duration should be within the range of 30–100 ms. Some authors even propose to use the pulse duration of 100 ms in all cases where the chronaxy is not known (Hayes, 1993). Most investigators report use of an amplitude within the patient's tolerance level of 15–35 mA (Valencic et al, 1986).

The ramp-up of the current should be three times longer than the ramp-down to increase the comfort for the patient. A monophasic pulse with an amplitude that gradually increases in an exponential fashion was first proposed over 40 years ago to stimulate denervated human muscle (Cummins, 1985; Kowarschik, 1952). If the denervated muscle is surrounded by innervated muscle, the gradual increase in amplitude may be needed to cause accommodation in the nearby innervated muscles, which are more sensitive to electrical stimulation. The on/off-time should include at least 5 seconds of rest between contractions with a preferred off-time of four to five times longer than the stimulation time (Thom, 1957).

The stimulating electrode (the cathode) should be positioned along the longitudinal fibers of the completely denervated muscle. A large dispersive pad should be located at a distant location. The response to stimulation will be sluggish rather than the brisk contraction observed when stimulating innervated muscle (Cummins, 1992). Multiple sites of stimulation will ensure that most of the denervated muscle fibers will contract despite a nonfunctional motor point (Hayes, 1988; Herbison et al, 1983).

In summary, it is important to realize that electrical stimulation of a partially denervated muscle is not beneficial and may impede reinnervation. If reinnervation is expected within 1–2 years, electrical stimulation to prevent muscle degeneration is not necessary. Electrical stimulation of a transplanted or reattached muscle is not recommended. Finally, the benefit of electrical stimulation to prevent atrophy in completely denervated muscle is beneficial for a limited time frame. Animal studies have shown that more than 6 weeks of electrical stimulation leads to atrophy of type I muscle fibers. Finally, the parameters for effective electrical stimulation of completely denervated human muscle remain controversial due to the paucity of well-controlled research studies outside of the laboratory animal model.

References

Albuquerque EX, McIsaac RJ: Fast and slow mammalian muscles after denervation. *Exp Neurol* 26:183, 1970.

Axelsson J, Thesleff S: A study of supersensitivity in denervated mammalian skeletal muscle. *J Physiol* 147:178, 1959.

Bowden RM, Gutmann E: Denervation and reinnervation of human voluntary muscle. *Brain* 67:273, 1944.

Brown MC, Holland RL: A central role for denervated tissue in causing nerve sprouting. *Nature* 282:714–726, 1979.

Cummins JP: Conservative management of peripheral nerve injuries utilizing selective electrical stimulation of denervated muscle with exponentially progressive current forms. *J Ortho Sports Phys Ther* 7:11–15, 1985.

Cummins JP: Electrical stimulation of denervated muscle, in MR Gersh, *Electrotherapy in Rehabilitation.* FA Davis, Philadelphia, 1992, p 270.

Girlanda PR, Dattola R, Vita G, et al: Effect of electrotherapy on denervated muscles in rabbits: An electrophysiological and morphological study. *Exp Neurol* 77:483–491, 1982.

Guth L, Kemerer VF, Samaras TA, et al: The roles of disuse and loss of neurotrophic function in denervation atrophy of skeletal muscle. *Exp Neurol* 73:20, 1981.

Gutmann E, Guttmann L: The effect of galvanic exercise on denervated and reinnervated muscles in the rabbit. *J Neurol Neurosurg Psychiat* 7:7, 1944.

Gutmann E, Zelena J: Morphological changes in the denervated muscle, in *Denervated Muscle*, E Gutmann (ed.). Prague, Publishing House of the Czechoslovak Academy of Sciences, 1962.

Hayes KW: Electrical stimulation and denervation: Proposed program and equipment limitations. *Top Acute Care Trauma Rehabil* 3(1):27–37, 1988.

Hayes KW: *Manual for Physical Agents*, 4th ed. Norwalk, CT, Appleton & Lange, 1993.

Herbison GJ, Jaweed MM, Ditunno JF: Exercise therapies in peripheral neuropathies. *Arch Phys Med Rehabil* 64:201–205, 1983.

Herbison GJ, Teng C, Gordon EE: Electrical stimulation of reinnervating rat muscle. *Arch Phys Med Rehabil* 54:156–160, 1973.

Jansen JKS, Lomo T, Nicolaysen K, et al: Hyperinnervation of skeletal muscle fibers: Dependence on muscle activity. *Science* 181(99):559–561, 1973.

Knowlton CC, Hines HM: Kinetics of muscle atrophy in different species. *Proc Soc Exp Biol Med* 35:394, 1936.

Kowarschik J: Exponential currents. *Br J Phys Med* 15:249, 1952.

Nix WA: The effect of low-frequency electrical stimulation on the denervated extensor digitorum longus muscle of the rabbit. *Acta Neurol Scand* 66:521–528, 1982.

Nix WA, Reichman H, Schroder MJ: Influence of direct low frequency stimulation on contractile properties of denervated fast-twitch rabbit muscle. *Pflugers Arch* 405:141, 1985.

Pachter BR, Eberstein A, Goodgold J: Electrical stimulation effect on denervated skeletal myofibers in rats: A light and electron microscopic study. *Arch Phys Med Rehabil* 63:427–430, 1982.

Schimrigk K, McLaughlin J, Grüninger W: The effect of electrical stimulation on the experimentally denervated rat muscle. *Scand J Rehabil Med* 9:55–60, 1977.

Spielholz NI: Electrical stimulation of denervated muscle, in RM Nelson, DP Currier, *Clinical Electrotherapy*, 2d ed. Appleton & Lange, Norwalk, CT, 1991, p 122.

Sunderland S: *Nerves and Nerve Injuries*, 2d ed. Edinburgh, Churchill Livingston, 1978.

Thom H: Treatment of paralyses with exponentially progressive currents. *Br J Phys Med* 20(3):49–56, 1957.

Valencic V, Vodovnik L, Stefancic M, Jelnikar T: Improved motor response due to chronic electrical stimulation of denervated tibialis anterior muscle in humans. *Muscle Nerve* 9:612–617, 1986.

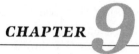

Electrical Stimulation of Abnormal Muscle Tone

Spasticity has been defined as a motor disorder characterized by a velocity-dependent increase in tonic stretch reflexes (muscle tone) with exaggerated tendon jerks (Lance, 1980). Clonus, the repetitive contraction of a hyperactive muscle in response to a quick stretch, is often present.

Neurologic insult to the brain or spinal cord often results in abnormally high muscle tone or spasticity. When the muscles are drawn into the shortened position at the elbow, knee, or hip, the term *flexor spasticity* is used. *Extensor spasticity* is used to describe the abnormal muscle tone that maintains the joints in a primarily extended position. Some injuries result in extensor spasticity of both lower extremities (diplegic cerebral palsy or lumbar spinal cord injury). Other injuries result in spasticity of the arm, leg, and trunk of one side of the body (hemiplegic cerebral palsy or stroke). More extensive involvement of the nervous system, following viral or bacterial infections or spinal cord injuries of the neck, result in abnormal muscle tone of all four extremities and the trunk.

In the spinal cord-injured patient, there is altered motor unit activity in response to either sensory or central inputs. This alteration results in a short period (about 3 months) of low muscle tone, followed by a period of flexor spasticity, and ultimately is followed by extensor spastic-

215

ity below the level of the lesion. The spasticity is characterized by cocontraction of the agonist and antagonistic muscles (Wiesendanger, 1991). The stroke patient experiences low muscle tone followed by a gradual increase in tone (Thilmann et al, 1991). The pattern of abnormal tone appears on the opposite side of the body as the location of the impaired circulation caused by the cerebral vascular accident (CVA). A typical pattern for the stroke patient is extensor tone in the affected lower extremity and flexor tone in the affected upper extremity. The affected side of the trunk may appear with either low or high muscle tone.

The orthopedic consequences of high muscle tone include joint contractures and dislocations (Samilson et al, 1972). Tendon releases, transfers, or both are often required in this population. Neurosurgery, such as the selective dorsal rhizotomy, has been shown to reduce lower extremity spasticity in the cerebral palsied child (Chicoine, 1997) Intrathecal infusion of Baclofen, an antispasticity drug, is effective in reducing abnormal muscle tone (Campbell et al, 1995; Gerszten et al, 1998; Shetter, 1993).

Treatment of the spasticity is indicated if the performance of self-care, gait, positioning, or transfers can be enhanced. In some cases, the extensor tone of the lower extremities is useful for standing, transfers, and gait and should not be reduced. Electrical stimulation, in conjunction with therapy, has been used to reduce spasticity for short periods of time, allowing the patient to experience normalized volitional movements and enhanced function (Hecox et al, 1994).

Electrical stimulation reduces abnormal tone through the induction of muscle fatigue, but may cause an adverse reaction of increased spasticity if pain is induced. (Benton et al, 1981; Stillwell, 1983). The ideal electrotherapy techniques vary according to the type of injury the patient has experienced. For example, repetitive electrical stimulation, causing habituation of the cutaneous sensation, can reduce the flexion reflex of the paraplegic patient when applied to the plantar surface of the foot (Dimitrijevic, 1970). A similar habituation pattern, with reduction in clonus, has been reported in a small sample of multiple sclerosis patients following subcutaneous nerve stimulation (Walker, 1982).

PROCEDURE 9–1

Electrical Stimulation to Reduce Abnormal Muscle Tone

Parameters	Settings
Current type/waveform	Symmetrical biphasic pulsed current if large muscles *or* asymmetrical biphasic pulsed current if small muscles, such as the hands or feet
Pulse duration	200–500 μs
Current amplitude	Maximum tolerable
Frequency	> 60 pps to produce tetany
On-time	2–10 seconds
Off-time	2–10 seconds
Treatment duration	15 minutes
Electrode configuration	*If small muscles:* one channel with two electrodes *If large muscles:* two channels with four electrodes Align over spastic muscles *or* antagonists

FCR
PL
FDS
FCU

Electrical stimulation to reduce abnormal muscle tone

SOURCE: Mehreteab TA: Effect of electrical stimulation on nerve and muscle tissues, in B Hecox, TA Mehreteab, J Weisberg: *Physical Agents: A Comprehensive Text for Physical Therapists.* Norwalk, CT, Appleton & Lange, 1994; p 287.

PROCEDURE 9–2

Electrical Stimulation to Reduce Abnormal Muscle Tone in Spinal Spasticity

Parameters	Settings
Current type/waveform	Symmetrical biphasic pulsed current if large muscles *or* asymmetrical biphasic pulsed current if small muscles, such as the hands or feet
Pulse duration	100–500 µs
Current amplitude	100 mA
Frequency	20–100 pps*
On-time	2.5 seconds
Off-time	2.5 seconds
Treatment duration	20 minutes
Electrode configuration	*If small muscles:* one channel with two electrodes *If large muscles:* two channels with four electrodes Align over spastic muscles *or* antagonists

FCR
PL
FDS
FCU

Electrical stimulation to reduce abnormal muscle tone

SOURCE: Vodovnik L, Stefanovska A, Bajd T: Effects of stimulation parameters on modification of spinal spasticity. *Med Biol Eng Comput* 25:439, 1987.

* 100 pps is more effective than 10 pps or 1000 pps in reducing abnormal muscle tone. Cycle duration is less critical, but 100 µs is preferred.

PROCEDURE 9–3

Reduction of Spasticity in Spinal Cord-injured Patients

Parameters	Settings
Current type/waveform	Rectangular monophasic pulsed current
Pulse duration	300 μs
Current amplitude	To tolerable sensory stimulation
Frequency	100 pps
Treatment duration	20 minutes
Electrode configuration	Two channels with four electrodes over quadriceps L3–L4 dermatome

OUTCOME: In six spinal cord-injured patients with moderate spasticity, 50% had marked decrease in tone as measured with the Pendulum test. This effect lasted less than 24 hours.

SOURCE: Bajd T, Gregoric M, Vodovnik L, Benko H: Electrical stimulation in treating spasticity resulting from spinal cord injury. Arch Phys Med Rehabil 66:515–517, 1985.

PROCEDURE 9–4

Electrical Stimulation in Conjunction With Isometric Exercise in Incomplete Spinal Cord-lesioned Patients

Parameters	Settings
Current type/waveform	Monophasic pulsed current
Pulse duration	400 µs
Mode	2.5 second train
Current amplitude	120–160 mA
Frequency	20 pps
On-time	2.5 seconds
Off-time	2.5 seconds
Treatment duration	20 minutes, 2 times a day (at least 4 hours apart) 6 days/week for 4–8 weeks. Treatment included isotonic quadriceps contraction against gravity during electrical stimulation. In addition, testing involved 20 minutes of resisted isometric contractions
Electrode configuration	2 channels: one to each leg so that the on-time alternates from the left to right legs Align over quadriceps

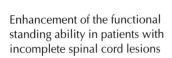

Enhancement of the functional standing ability in patients with incomplete spinal cord lesions

PROCEDURE 9–4

Continued

OTHER: Patients sat in wheelchairs or were supine with their legs elevated during application of electrical stimulation.

OUTCOME: This electrotherapy protocol, in conjunction with isometric and isotonic muscle contractions, improved the muscle tone of the knee extensors, which assisted the spinal cord-injured patient's functional standing ability.

SOURCE: Robinson CJ, Kett NA, Bolam JM: Spasticity in spinal cord-injured patients: 2. Initial measures and long-term effects of surface electrical stimulation. *Arch Phys Med Rehabil* 69:862–868, 1988.

PROCEDURE 9–5

Stimulation of the Antagonistic Muscle to Reduce Abnormal Muscle Tone

Parameters	Settings
Current type/waveform	Symmetrical biphasic pulsed current *or* asymmetrical biphasic pulsed current
Pulse duration	200–500 μs
Duty cycle	50%
Current amplitude	To produce tolerable muscle contraction
Frequency	> 30 pps to produce tetanic contraction
On-time	2–10 seconds
Off-time	10 seconds
Treatment duration	15–20 minutes
Electrode configuration	Align over antagonist muscles

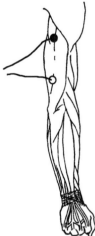

Electrical stimulation of the antagonistic muscle to reduce abnormal muscle tone of the agonist

OTHER: This protocol should be followed by a vigorous bout of range-of-motion exercises.

SOURCE: Levine MG, Knott M, Kabat H: Relaxation of spasticity by electrical stimulation of antagonist muscles. *Arch Phys Med* 33:668–673, 1952.

PROCEDURE 9–6

Sensory Stimulation of Antagonist Muscle in Hemiparetic Patients

Parameters	Settings
Current type/waveform	Asymmetrical biphasic continuous current rectangular waveform
Cycle duration	125 μs
Current amplitude	2 times the sensory threshold
Frequency	100 Hz
Treatment duration	45 minutes
Electrode configuration	Align over nerve to antagonist muscle
	Example: stimulate the peroneal nerve to treat plantar flexor spasticity

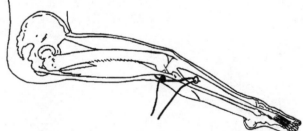

Electrical stimulation at the sensory level to reduce spasticity in the patient afflicted by cerebral vascular accident, head injury, or cerebral palsy

OUTCOME: This procedure resulted in a 1 hour reduction in the deep tendon reflex (DTR) magnitude, a measure of the degree of spasticity. When this electrotherapy protocol was used to induce tetanic contractions in the muscles of patients afflicted by cerebral vascular accident (CVA), traumatic brain injury (TBI), or cerebral palsy (CP), abnormal muscle tone was reduced up to several hours following cessation of the electrical stimulation.

SOURCE: Hui-Chan CWY, Levine MG: Stretch reflex latencies in spastic hemiparetic subjects are prolonged after transcutaneous electrical nerve stimulation. Can J Neurol Sci 20:47–106, 1993.

PROCEDURE 9–7

Electrical Stimulation of the Antagonistic Muscle in the Patient After a Cerebral Vascular Accident (CVA)

Parameters	Settings
Current type/waveform	Monophasic pulsed current, square wave
Pulse duration	50 μs
Current amplitude	Increase to a level that does not produce overflow to adjacent muscles
Frequency	50 pps
On-time	2 seconds
Off-time	2 seconds
Treatment duration	10 minutes/day × 8–17 treatments
Electrode configuration	Align active electrode over motor point of the antagonistic muscle

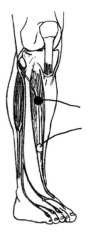

Electrical stimulation of the cerebral vascular accident (CVA) patient's dorsiflexor muscles to reduce spasticity in the plantar flexor muscles

OUTCOME: In 96 hemiplegic patients, 90% experienced decreased spasticity lasting from 10 minutes to 2 hours.

SOURCE: Alfieri V: Electrical treatment of spasticity: Reflex tonic activity in hemiplegic patients and selected specific electrostimulation. *Scand J Rehab Med* 14:177–182, 1982.

PROCEDURE 9–8

Antagonistic Stimulation of Spastic Hand Muscles in Cerebral Vascular Accident (CVA) Patients

Parameters	Settings
Current type/waveform	Monophasic pulsed current
Pulse duration	200 μs
Current amplitude	To sustain isotonic contraction through full range of motion
Frequency	33 pps
On-time	7 seconds
Off-time	10 seconds
Treatment duration	15 minutes twice daily initially; then 30 minutes three times daily for 4 weeks
Electrode configuration	Align over antagonistic muscle

Electrical stimulation of the antagonistic muscles to reduce spasticity in the cerebral vascular accident (CVA) patient's wrist and fingers

SOURCE: Baker LL, Yeh C, Wilson D, Waters RL: Electrical stimulation of wrist and fingers for hemiplegic patients. Phys Ther 59:1495–1499, 1979.

PROCEDURE 9–9

Reciprocal Stimulation of Spastic and Antagonistic Muscles in Spinal Cord-injured Patients

Parameters	Settings
Current type/waveform	Asymmetrical biphasic pulsed current
Pulse duration	300 μs
Current amplitude	100 mA
Frequency	30 pps
On-time	5 seconds
Off-time	5 seconds
Treatment duration	30 minutes
Electrode configuration	Align over hamstrings of limb one and quadriceps of limb two

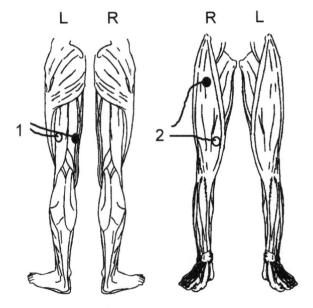

Reciprocal stimulation of the spastic and antagonistic muscles in the spinal cord-injured patient's legs

PROCEDURE 9–9

Continued

Parameters	Settings

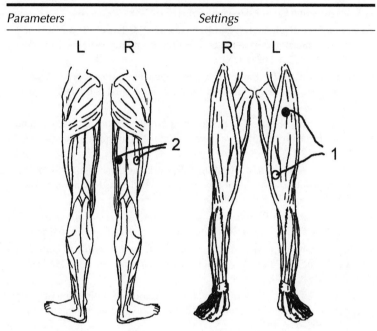

Reciprocal stimulation of the spastic and antagonistic muscles in the spinal cord-injured patient's legs

> After first 30 minute session align electrodes over quadriceps of limb one and hamstrings of limb two and repeat stimulation protocol

OUTCOME: Reciprocal pattern of antispasticity stimulation is not superior to either agonist or antagonistic stimulation approaches in this study with 7 spinal cord-injured patients. The authors reported decreased spasticity for 10 minutes to 2 hours after cessation of electrical stimulation.

SOURCE: Vodovnik L, Bowman BR, Hufford P: Effects of electrical stimulation on spinal spasticity. *Scand J Rehab Med* 16:29–34, 1984.

References

Benton LA, Baker LL, Bowman BR, Waters RL: *Functional Electrical Stimulation: A Practical Clinical Guide.* Rancho Los Amigos Rehabilitation Engineering Center, Downey, CA, 1981.

Campbell SK, Almeida GL, Penn RD, Corcos DM: The effects of intrathecally administered baclofen on function in patients with spasticity. *Phys Ther* 75(5):352–362, 1995.

Chicoine MR, Park TS, Kaufman BA: Selective dorsal rhizotomy and rates of orthopedic surgery in children with spastic cerebral palsy. *J Neurosurg* 86:34–39, 1997.

Dimitrijevic MR, Nathan PW: Studies of spasticity in man: 4. Changes in flexion reflex with repetitive cutaneous stimulation in spinal man. *Brain* 93:743, 1970.

Gerszten PC, Albright AL, Johnstone GF: Intrathecal baclofen infusion and subsequent orthopedic surgery in patients with spastic cerebral palsy. *J Neurosurg* 88:1009–1013, 1998.

Hecox B, Mehreteab TA, Weisberg J: *Physical Agents: A Comprehensive Text for Physical Therapists.* Norwalk, CT, Appleton & Lange, 1994; p 286.

Lance JW: Symposium synopsis, in *Spasticity: Disordered Motor Control*, RG Feldman, RR Young, WP Koella (eds.). Chicago, Year Book Medical Publishers, 1980; pp 485–494.

Samilson RL, Tsou P, Aamoth G, et al: Dislocation and subluxation of the hip in cerebral palsy: Pathogenesis, natural history and management. *JBJS* 54-A:863–873, 1972.

Shetter AG: Intrathecal baclofen in the treatment of spasticity of spinal origin: Rationale, surgical techniques, and patient monitoring. *Perspect Neurol Surg* 4:109–122, 1993.

Stillwell GK: *Therapeutic Electricity and Ultraviolet Radiation*, 3rd ed. Baltimore, Williams & Wilkins, 1983; p 160.

Thilmann AF, Fellows SJ, Garms E: The mechanism of spastic muscle hypertonus variation in reflex gain over the time course of spasticity. *Brain* 114:233–244, 1991.

Walker JB: Modulation of spasticity: Prolonged suppression of a spinal reflex by electrical stimulation. *Science* 216:203, 1982.

Wiesendanger M: Neurophysiological basis of spasticity, in *Neurosurgery for Spasticity*, M Sindou, R Abbott, Y Kerevel (eds.). New York, Springer-Verlag, 1991; pp 15–19.

CHAPTER 10

Electrical Stimulation of the Spinal Cord-injured Patient

Following a spinal cord injury (SCI), a decrease in muscle bulk, a reduction in force, and an increase in fatigue of the affected muscle occurs. Electrical stimulation of the muscles has been shown to increase muscle endurance and prevent the losses in lean body mass associated with an acute SCI. In addition, electrical stimulation of the affected muscles has been reported to improve circulation, reduce abnormal muscle tone, increase range of motion, and increase the spinal cord-injured patient's sensory awareness. Electrical stimulation, without inducing pain, should be provided twice a day to strengthen the hip and knee extensors as soon as possible after an SCI. Electrical stimulation is then used to initiate and maintain standing of the SCI patient. The patient's muscle endurance and ability to overcome jack-knifing will determine the standing duration, which is, on average, 10–20 minutes. Once the SCI patient masters static standing, progression to functional dynamic standing for activities of daily living and gait training are begun with the assistance of electrical stimulation systems.

Muscle fatigue in the spinal cord-injured patient receiving electrical stimulation is greater than the fatigue experienced with volitional muscle contraction because the order of muscle fiber recruitment is reversed. Fatigue can be alleviated with the use of sequential electrical stimulation of muscle groups coupled with adequate recovery time between stimulation. Sequential electrical stimulation is a complex issue requiring regulation of muscle force, control over the resultant joint position, and coordination of synergistic and multijoint muscle contractions.

Functional surface electrical stimulation using electrode garments allows specific sequencing for stimulation of eight muscles per limb and rapid and secure application of the electrodes. The garments contain pockets and built-in wires for rapid and secure application of the multiple stimulation electrodes. For instance, garments used to assist the spinal cord-injured patient with standing and walking have secured electrodes positioned over the quadriceps and peroneal nerve (Patterson et al, 1990).

Electrode garments designed to assist the spinal cord-injured patient in maintaining muscle mass and bone density through the riding of a stationary bike are commercially available (Bioflex Electrode Garment, Therapeutic Alliance, Inc., 333 North Broad Street, Fairborn, OH 45324); and Stimwear Electrode Garment, also from Therapeutic Alliance, Inc.). In addition, functional electrical stimulation cycle ergometers (REGYS or ERGYS; Therapeutic Alliances, Inc.), use an electrode garment and computer software to stimulate the quadriceps, hamstrings, and gluteal muscles sequentially (Petrofsky, Phillips, Stafford, 1984; Ragnarsson et al, 1988). Sensors provide on-line feedback to allow automatic adjustment of the stimulation parameters. The aerobic cycling program for the SCI patient should not be initiated if there is the presence of autonomic dysreflexia; pressure ulcers; fractures; heterotopic ossification; joint subluxation; demand-type pacemaker; heart disease; ailments where high fever, high blood pressure, or high heart rate are present; severe osteoporosis; limited range of motion in the hips or knees; denervated muscle; severe muscle spasticity; cancer or infection in the area; history of hip disarticulation; or muscle disease (Therapeutic Alliances Inc).

Electrically induced cycling has been shown to significantly increase circulation, cardiovascular work performance, and maximal oxygen uptake of the spinal cord-injured patient (Hooker et al, 1995; Mohr et al, 1997; Nash et al, 1996). Initially, patients perform unloaded cycling for 5 minutes. In each succeeding session, the cycling duration is increased until the patient is able to pedal for 30 continuous minutes. Once the patient can complete two consecutive 30 minute sessions at a given resistance, the workload is increased by 6.1 watts (1/8 kp). If the patient fatigues during the training session, performing less than 35 revolutions per minute (rpm), the workload is reduced to the previous level, and exercise continues for a total of 30 minutes (Hooker et al, 1995).

In static standing, continuous maximal stimulation of the knee and hip extensor muscles is used to lock the knee safely. This technique, however, results in ischemia and fatigue of the quadriceps and, therefore, limits standing time. (Mulder, 1992; Nuzik, 1986; Petrofsky, Phillips, Sandford, 1984).

The paraplegic patient typically ambulates with forearm crutches and orthotics with knee locks. The energy cost and resultant muscle fatigue in the upper extremities limits the amount of time for ambulation. The paraplegic patient with good trunk control can stand with the aid of electrical stimulation to the knee extensor muscles in conjunction with the use of a walker and ankle-foot orthoses (AFOs).

There are a number of hybrid systems that use a rolling walker, orthoses, and electrical stimulation to assist the paraplegic patient in functional upright activities and reciprocal gait, such as the Reciprocal Gait Orthoses (RGO) (Douglas et al, 1983); the Oswestry Parawalker Orthosis (Stallard et al, 1986; Butler, 1987); the Akita Knee Joint System (Kagaya et al, 1996); and the Parastep System (Sigmedics, Inc, One Northfield Plaza Suite 111, Northfield IL, 60093) (Gallien et al, 1995; Graupe and Kohn, 1994). Rolling walkers with a microprocessor-based electrical stimulation device allow the paraplegic patient to activate the stimulation sequence with thumb switches on the handles of the walker. Some of the systems are programmed such that when the patient activates the left thumb switch, the left quadriceps muscle group and the right hamstrings muscle group will receive simultaneous electrical stimulation. Alternatively, some systems stimulate knee flexion by using the flexion withdrawal reflex. When the paraplegic patient presses both the left and the right thumb switch, electrical stimulation of the left and right hip and knee extensor muscles occur. This bilateral activation allows the patient to stand up using the walker for support (Douglas et al, 1983; Thoumie et al, 1995). It should be noted that hybrid systems are designed for short-distance ambulation of the spinal cord-injured patient. Community ambulation of the paraplegic patient using a hybrid system is an unreasonable expectation (Winchester et al, 1994).

In the *open* loop control configuration, a predetermined pattern of stimulation, is provided to the muscles upon pressing the activation switch on the walker. In practice, these systems do not provide enough muscle contraction to achieve the desired movement. Alternatively, the predetermined stimulation pattern may provide too much contraction of the muscles and result in excessive musculoskeletal stresses.

Development of the *closed* loop control configuration is still under investigation. In this system, information about the force of movement and position of the limb are fed back to the stimulator. Adjustment of the output is made to meet the time-specific functional requirements.

For the incomplete spinal cord-injured patient with normal trunk control, the heel switch is often used to aid in ambulation while increasing muscle force and reducing muscle fatigue (Liberson et al, 1961; Rochester et al, 1995). The heel switch is located in the shoe and triggers dorsiflexion of the foot when the heel is raised off the floor. Alternatively, a pressure sensor over the crutch handle or a clinician-controlled hand-held switch could be used to activate the sequence of electrical stimulation during gait (Andrews, 1988; Kralj, 1989).

For tetraplegic patients, a transcutaneous multichannel system may be applied to assist in functional arm movements (Naito et al, 1994; Nathan, 1984; Nathan, 1989). This system, which is capable of generating and coordinating fine motor control, requires careful technical placement of the electrodes on 12 muscles. Fifteen muscles are activated to generate finger, thumb, wrist, and elbow movements (Nathan, 1990). For most electrical stimulation systems used on the tetraplegic patients surgically implanted electrodes are needed.

Implanted electrodes have been used clinically since the 1970s to improve the function of the neurologically impaired patient (Marsolais and Kobetic, 1987; Peckham and Mortiner, 1977; Smith et al, 1994). Implanted electrodes overcome the shortcomings of surface electrodes (donning/doffing times, variation in deep muscle activation, and high cutaneous sensory stimulation). Research continues to evaluate the muscle tissue response to implanted electrodes over extended time frames.

Implanted electrodes have also been used to control lower extremity movements using a closed loop system with 26 channels of electrical stimulation; however, the movements are uncoordinated and often require repositioning of the limb to prevent a fall or serious injury (Marsolais and Kobetic, 1987).

The clinician applying other electrical stimulation must thoroughly evaluate the patient for subcutaneous devices (such as the phrenic nerve stimulator), anterior sacral root stimulation (for the treatment of neurogenic bladder dysfunction), transabdominal electrical stimulation, or pumps (such as the Baclofen pump for spasticity control), since the application of electrical stimulation may be contraindicated. The electrical stimulation systems should not be used on paraplegic patients with cardiac demand pacemakers, cancer, infection, skin disease, edema, inflammation, phlebitis, thrombophlebitis, varicose veins in the area of electrode placement, severe scoliosis or osteoporosis, irreversible contractures, or autonomic dysreflexia. Precautions should be taken if electrical stimulation is used on patients with suspected heart or pulmonary disease, seizure disorder, vision or hearing impairments that interfere with training, bleeding or bruising disorders, hypersensitivity to electrical conductive medium, tape, or electrical stimulation. Safety has not been established for the use of electrode garments or multichannel hybrid systems on children or pregnant patients (Sigmedics, Inc, One Northfield Plaza, Suite 111, Northfield IL, 60093).

PROCEDURE 10–1

Electrical Stimulation of the Forearm and Hand Muscles of C4–C5 Tetraplegic Patients

Parameters	Settings
Current	Monophasic pulsed current, square waveform
Pulse duration	300 μs
Current amplitude	Increased in 1 mA increments to a maximum of 60 mA
Frequency	30 pps
On-time	1 second burst
Off-time	700 μs between pulses, 1 second rest between bursts
Electrode configuration	The extensor pollicis longus (EPL) overflowed to the extensor digitorum (ED) and extensor indicis (EI). The extensor carpi radialis brevis (ECRB) overflowed to the ED. The extensor pollicis brevis (EPB) and abductor pollicis longus (APL) were activated simultaneously. All of the following muscles were individually activated: EPL, extensor carpi ulnaris (ECU), flexor digitorum superficialis (FDS), flexor carpi ulnaris (FCU), flexor digitorum profundus (FDP), flexor pollicis longus (FPL), first interosseus, second interosseus, and triceps.
Patient position	Upper limb is supported in a functional midrange position with the upper arm flexed, pronated, and abducted to 30°

OTHER: A bipolar search probe with two rubber 6 × 14 mm electrodes, arranged colinearly with an adjustable interelectrode distance, is used to find maximal response for cathode and anode.

PROCEDURE 10–1

Continued

OUTCOME: The index finger was the most difficult to stimulate, but it could be activated for prehension using the motor points for the FDS on the medial side of the muscle with overflow to the flexor carpi radialis (FCR). The EPL required several milliamperes more current amplitude than the other finger extensors for the release of objects. Fine control is lost if high gripping forces are required. Unacceptable overflow occurs when the wrist flexors are stimulated to the limit. Similarly, unacceptable overflow to the FPL and then the FDS occurs when the EPB and EPL are overstimulated.

SOURCE: Nathan RH: FNS of the upper limb: Targeting the forearm muscles for surface stimulation. *Med Biol Eng Comput* 28:249–256, 1990.

PROCEDURE 10-2

Voice Activated Electrical Stimulation for Arm and Hand Function in the C4 Tetraplegic Patient

Parameters	Settings
Current	Monophasic pulsed current, square waveform
Pulse duration	300–700 µs
Current amplitude	Increased in 1 mA increments to a maximum of 40 mA
Frequency	15 pps (to prevent fatigue) or up to 50 pps when recruitment of deeper muscle fibers needed
Treatment duration	4 hours
Electrode configuration	12 carbonized rubber electrode pairs (5 × 17 mm) are held in place by an elastic mesh. The following muscles are stimulated: trapezius, rhomboid, triceps, biceps, ECU, ECRB, FCR, EPL, EPB, ED, FDP, FDS, FPL, thenar group, and the first interosseus
Voice recognition	Voice Input Module, CA Smarthome.com, Inc. 17171 Daimler St Irvine, CA 92614-5508 (800) 762-7846

OTHER: A suspension system was used to control the forearm.

OUTCOME: Preprogrammed movement sequences, with the amplitude and pulse frequency for each muscle or channel, can be stored for use at a later date.

SOURCE: Nathan RH: An FNS-based system for generating upper limb function in the C4 quadriplegic. Med Biol Eng Comput 27:549–556, 1989.

PROCEDURE 10–3

Electrical Stimulation to Induce Standing in the T5–T6 Spinal Lesioned Patient

Parameters	Settings
Current	Monophasic pulsed current, rectangular waveform
Pulse duration	300 µs
Current amplitude	The maximum stimulation amplitude was defined as the value sufficient to stretch the leg against an external leg load that equaled half the trunk load of an average subject (about 20 kg)
Ramp	Based on feedback from angular velocity and angle of knee
Frequency	20 pps
On-time	Approximately 30 seconds but based on feedback from angular velocity and angle of knee
Off-time	5 minutes
Treatment duration	60 minutes (for 10 standing sessions of 30 seconds each) for 6 months
Electrode configuration	4 × 7 cm rubber electrodes over the rectus femoris motor point and near the patella
Electrogoniometer	An electrogoniometer was used to measure the knee angle and was sampled at 100 Hz and low-pass-filtered with a digital first-order filter at 15 Hz. Angular velocity was calculated digitally from the knee angle intersample difference and smoothed by a digital third-order, low-pass filter at 15 Hz

(*continued*)

PROCEDURE 10–3
Continued

OTHER: Patients had normal excitability of the quadriceps muscle and were trained with weight lifting up to 5 kg for 30 minute and low-load cycling 30–60 minutes twice a week.

SOURCES:

Mulder AJ, Boom HBK, Hermens HJ, Zilvold G: Artificial-reflex stimulation for FES-induced standing with minimum quadriceps force. *Med Biol Eng Comput* 28:483–488, 1990.

Mulder AJ, Veltink PH, Boom HBK: On/off control in FES-induced standing up: A model study and experiments. *Med Biol Eng Comput* 30:205–212, 1992.

PROCEDURE 10-4

Electrode Garment to Assist the Spinal Cord-injured Patient in Standing and Stepping

Parameters	Settings
Pulse duration	350 μs
Current amplitude	Up to 120 mA for quadriceps stimulation, 80 mA for peroneal nerve stimulation
Frequency	40 Hz
Electrode configuration	Two channels with 4 cm electrodes for bilateral peroneal nerve stimulation (in popliteal fossa behind the head of the fibula), two channels with 50 cm² electrodes for quadriceps stimulation, two channels for gluteus medius and gluteus maximus stimulation, and two channels for stimulation of the tibialis anterior

Location of the stimulation sites within the electrode garment to assist the spinal cord-injured patient with hip extension and knee flexion

(continued)

PROCEDURE 10–4

Continued

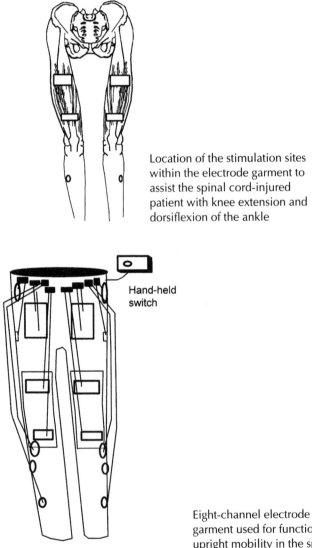

Location of the stimulation sites within the electrode garment to assist the spinal cord-injured patient with knee extension and dorsiflexion of the ankle

Hand-held switch

8-channel electrode garment

Eight-channel electrode garment used for functional upright mobility in the spinal cord-injured person

PROCEDURE 10–4

Continued

Parameters	Settings
Electrode garment	BioStim Trend Corp, 14851 NW 27th Ave, Opa Locka, FL 33054
Hand-held switch	Hand-held stimulation activates the flexor withdrawal reflex for step while interrupting the quadriceps stimulation on that side

OUTCOME: All patients used crutches or a walker for stability. Two patients (T4 and C7) were able to stand for 30 minutes and walk up to 60 m at a rate of 8.7 m/minute. Long leg braces were not needed, but an AFO was needed in some situations.

SOURCE: Patterson RP, Lockwood JS, Dykstra KK: A functional electric stimulation system using an electrode garment. *Arch Phys Med Rehabil* 71:340–342, 1990.

PROCEDURE 10–5

Stimulation of the Tibialis Anterior After Spinal Cord Injury to Increase Fatigue Resistance

Parameters	Settings
Current	Pulsed current, square wave
Pulse duration	2 ms, 80 pulses in a 25 ms pulse train
Amplitude	To maximum twitch
Frequency	20 pps
Duty cycle	50%
On-time	5 seconds
Off-time	5 seconds
Treatment duration	6 week periods of (1) 15 minutes/day, (2) 45 minutes/day, (3) 2 hours/day, (4) 8 hours/day, and (5) 45 minutes/day, for a total of 30 weeks
Electrode configuration	4.5 cm² with the cathode over the motor point of the tibialis anterior muscle and the anode placed about 9 cm distally
Unit	Respond II (formerly of Medtronic, currently with EMPI) EMPI, Inc 599 Cardigan Rd St Paul, MN 55126-3965 (800) 328-2536

OUTCOME: Five adults, ages 22–38 years, with complete motor loss spinal cord injury (C6–T4), were enrolled in the study 2–11 years postinjury. Stimulation at 2 hours/day appears to have been sufficient to increase the fatigue resistance of the affected muscle to a level close to a normal value.

SOURCE: Stein RB, Gordon T, Jefferson J, et al: Optimal stimulation of paralyzed muscle after human spinal cord injury. J Appl Physiol 72(4):1393–1400, 1992.

PROCEDURE 10-6

Electrical Stimulation to Control the Swing Phase of Paraplegic Gait

Parameters	Settings
Pulse duration	Maximal attainable without undesired "spillover" to other muscles
Burst duration	Hamstrings: 120 ms; hip flexors: 200–400 ms; quadriceps: 160–200 ms
Amplitude	Maximal attainable without undesired "spillover" to other muscles
Frequency	Hip flexors: 50 Hz; hamstrings and quadriceps: 25 Hz
On-time	Determined relative to trigger instant
Off-time	Interpulse interval was 40 ms for the quadriceps and 20 ms for the hamstrings
Treatment duration	30 minutes/day
Electrode configuration	5 × 9 cm used on three muscle groups: (1) hip flexors with cathode in the groin fold on the lateral surface and the anode in the groin fold slightly distal and medial, (2) quadriceps with the cathode over the motor point for the rectus femoris and the anode over the vastus medialis, and (3) midline of the posterior thigh with the cathode at midthigh and the anode slightly proximal to the popliteal fossa

(continued)

PROCEDURE 10–6

Continued

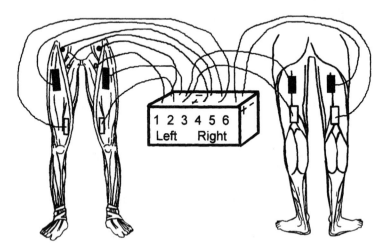

Location of the stimulation sites to assist the paraplegic person with hip flexion and knee control during the swing phase of gait

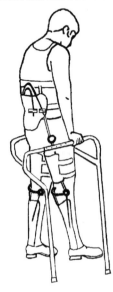

Electrical stimulation with a reciprocating gait orthosis walker to assist the T5–T6 paraplegic patient in ambulation

PROCEDURE 10–6

Continued

Parameters	Settings
Sequence of stimulation	Hip flexors, hamstrings, quadriceps

OTHER: Standing frame, modified advanced reciprocating gait orthosis, and goniometers at the hip and knee were used.

OUTCOME: Two complete T5–T6 paraplegic patients were enrolled in the study. One patient experienced muscle spasms resulting in knee extension throughout most of the swing phase. In the other patient, knee extension occurred too early or too late due to excessive hip flexion. Toe clearance was difficult for both subjects at times. Hip flexors fatigued faster than the other muscle groups due to the higher frequency of stimulation required.

SOURCE: Franken HM, Veltinik PH, Baardman G, et al: Cycle-to-cycle control of swing phase of paraplegic gait induced by surface electrical stimulation. Med Biol Eng Comput 33:440–451, 1995.

PROCEDURE 10-7

Electrical Stimulation
of the Paraplegic Patient to
Assist in Standing and Stepping

Parameters	Settings
Current	Pulsed current, rectangular waveform
Pulse duration	300 μs
Amplitude	200 mA from a 120 V source
Frequency	24 Hz
Treatment duration	10–30 minutes twice a day for 10–30 days
Electrode configuration	Two channels for the quadriceps and one channel for the flexor withdrawal reflex for a total of six channels per patient; 4.5 × 4.5 cm cathodes (–) on the vastus lateralis and gluteus medius with anodes on the rectus femoris and vastus lateralis. Flexor withdrawal achieved with a 3.5 × 4.5 cm anode (+) approximately 4 cm below the head of the fibula and the cathode about 5 cm distal to this

Location of the six channel electrical stimulation electrodes used to assist the paraplegic patient in standing and stepping

OUTCOME: Four spinal cord-injured patients, 28–48 years of age, were enrolled in the study at 7–30 years postinjury. Use of electrical stimulation with a walker enabled paraplegics to stand with 40–70% weightbearing through the feet and to take primitive steps at a velocity of 7–10 cm/second.

SOURCE: Mizrahi J, Braun A, Najenson T, Graupe D: Quantitative weightbearing and gait evaluation of paraplegics using functional electrical stimulation. *Med Biol Eng Comput* 23:101–107, 1985.

PROCEDURE 10–8

Electrical Stimulation of an Incomplete C7 Spinal Cord-injured Patient to Assist in Gait

Parameters	Settings
Current	Monophasic pulsed current, rectangular waveform
Pulse duration	300 μs
Amplitude	70–90 V (due to preserved pain sensations)
Frequency	20 pps
On/off-time	Knee extension was initiated when the hand switch was released and stopped when the hand switch was pressed. Ankle dorsiflexion was initiated when the crutch sensor was pressed and stopped when the hand switch was pressed. Thus, pressing the hand switch marked the end of stance and the beginning of the swing phase. The flexion reflex for limb clearance in swing was initiated when the hand switch was pressed (with simultaneous cessation of knee extension and dorsiflexion)
Electrode configuration	*Channel one:* 6 × 4 cm electrodes with water-soaked gauze as the conducting medium are placed over the knee extensors
	Channel two: A 2 cm electrode is placed over the peroneal nerve near the popliteal fossa with the second 2 cm electrode behind the fibular head (above the trunk of the superficial peroneal nerve)
	Channel three: 6 cm electrodes are used to stimulate ankle plantar flexors

(*continued*)

PROCEDURE **10-8**

Continued

Parameters	Settings

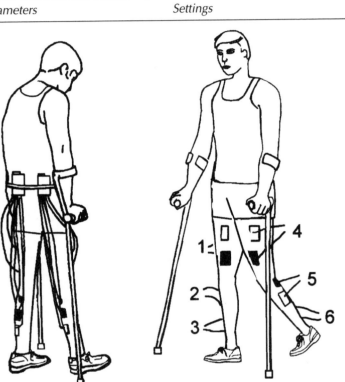

Posterior view of channels two and three used to stimulate knee flexion and ankle plantar flexion during gait of the incomplete C7 spinal cord-injured patient

Anterior view of the electrical stimulation sites used to assist the incomplete C7 spinal cord-injured patient in gait

Unit

Advanced CMOS Logic
Texas Instruments, Inc
12500 TI Blvd
Dallas, TX 75243-4136
(800) 336-5236

PROCEDURE 10–8
Continued

OTHER: Gait control events are obtained from leading of the Lofstrand crutch sensor, pressing of the hand switch, and releasing the hand switch.

OUTCOME: An 18-year-old tetraparetic patient was enrolled in the study. The patient had voluntary control of one lower limb with sufficient strength for safe standing. Three-channel electrical stimulation was applied only to the affected limb.

SOURCE: Bajd T, Munih M, Dralj A, et al: Voluntary commands for FES-assisted walking in incomplete SCI subjects. *Med Biol Eng Comput* 33:334–337, 1995.

References

Andrews BJ, Baxendale RH, Barnett R, et al: Hybrid FES orthosis incorporating closed loop control and sensory feedback. *J Biodmed Eng* 10:189–195, 1988.

Butler PB, Major R: The Para Walker: A rational approach to the provision of reciprocal ambulation for paraplegic patients . . . formerly hip guidance orthosis. *Physiotherapy* 73(8):393–397, 1987.

Douglas R, Larson PF, D'Ambrosia R, McCall RE: The LSU reciprocating gait orthosis. *Orthopedics* 6:834–838, 1983.

Gallien P, Brissot R, Eyssette M, et al: Restoration of gait by functional electrical stimulation for spinal cord injured patients. *Paraplegia* 33:660–664, 1995.

Graupe D, Kohn KH: A critical review of EMG controlled electrical stimulation in paraplegics. *CRC Crit Rev Biomed Eng* 15:187–210, 1994.

Hooker SP, Scremin E, Mutton DL, et al: Peak and submaximal physiologic responses following electrical stimulation leg cycle ergometer training. *J Rehabil Res Dev* 32(4):361–366, 1995.

Kagaya H, Shimada Y, Sato K, et al: An electrical knee lock system for functional electrical stimulation. *Arch Phys Med Rehabil* 77:870–873, 1996.

Kralj A, Bajd T: *Functional Electrical Stimulation: Standing and Walking After Spinal Cord Injury.* Boca Raton, FL, CRC Press, 1989.

Liberson WT, Homquest HJ, Scott D, Dow M: Functional electrotherapy: Stimulation of the peroneal nerve synchronized with the swing phase of the gait of hemiplegic patients. *Arch Phys Med Rehabil* 42:101–105, 1961.

Marsolais EB, Kobetic R: Functional electrical stimulation for walking in paraplegia. *JBJS* 69-A:728–733, 1987.

Mohr T, Andersen J, Biering-Sørensen F, et al: Long term adaptation to electrically induced cycle training in severe spinal cord injured individuals. *Spinal Cord* 35:1–6, 1997.

Mulder AJ, Veltink PH, Boom HBK: On/off control in FES-induced standing up: A model study and experiments. *Med Biol Eng Comput* 30:205–212, 1992.

Naito A, Yajima M, Fukamachi H, et al: Functional electrical stimulation (FES) to the biceps brachii for controlling forearm supination in the paralyzed upper extremity. *Tohoku J Exp Med* 173(2):269–273, 1994.

Nash MS, Montalvo BM, Applegate B: Lower extremity blood flow and responses to occlusion ischemia differ in exercise-trained and sedentary tetraplegic persons. *Arch Phys Med Rehabil* 77:1260–1265, 1996.

Nathan R: The development of a computerized upper limb electrical stimulation system. *Orthopedics* 7:1170–1180, 1984.

Nathan RH: An FNS-based system for generating upper limb function in the C4 quadriplegic. *Med Biol Eng Comput* 27:549–556, 1989.

Nathan RH: FNS of the upper limb: Targeting the forearm muscles for surface stimulation. *Med Biol Eng Comput* 28:249–256, 1990.

Nuzik S, Lamb R, VanSant A, Hirt S: Sit-to-stand movement pattern: A kinematic study. *Phys Ther* 66:1708–1713, 1986.

Patterson RP, Lockwood JS, Dykstra DD: A functional electric stimulation system using an electrode garment. *Arch Phys Med Rehabil* 71:340–342, 1990.

Peckham PH, Mortimer JT: Restoration of hand function in the quadriplegic through electrical stimulation, in *Functional Electrical Stimulation: Application in Neural Prostheses*, FT Hambrecht, JB Reswick (eds.). New York, Marcel Dekker, 1977; pp 83–95.

Petrofsky JS, Phillips CA: The use of functional electrical stimulation for rehabilitation of spinal cord injured patients. *Cent Nerv Syst Trauma* 1:57–74, 1984.

Petrofsky JS, Phillips CA, Stafford DE: Closed-loop control for restoration of movement in paralyzed muscle. *Orthopedics* 7:1289–1302, 1984.

Ragnarsson KT, Pollack SF, O'Daniel W, et al: Clinical evaluation of computerized functional electrical stimulation after spinal cord injury: A multicenter pilot study. *Arch Phys Med Rehabil* 69:672–677, 1988.

Rochester L, Chandler CS, Johnson MA, et al: Influence of electrical stimulation of the tibialis anterior muscle in paraplegic subjects: 1. Contractile properties. *Paraplegia* 33(8):437–449, 1995.

Smith BT, Betz RR, Mulcahey MJ, et al: Reliability of percutaneous intramuscular electrodes for upper extremity functional neuromuscular stimulation in adolescents with C5 tetraplegia. *Arch Phys Med Rehabil* 75(9):939–945, 1994.

Stallard J, Major RE, Poiner R, et al: Engineering design considerations of the ORLAU ParaWalker and FES hybrid system. *Eng Med* 15:123–129, 1986.

Thoumie P, Perrouin-Verbe B, Le Claire G, et al: Restoration of functional gait in paraplegic patients with the RGO-II hybrid orthosis: A multicentre controlled study: Clinical evaluation. *Paraplegia* 33:647–653, 1995.

Winchester P, Carollo JJ, Habasevich R: Physiologic costs of reciprocal gait in FES assisted walking. *Paraplegia* 32:680–686, 1994.

CHAPTER 11

Electrical Stimulation of the Stroke Patient

Immediately following an upper motor neuron lesion, such as a cerebrovascular accident (CVA) or stroke, the affected extremities become flaccid in approximately 90% of the patients (Poulin de Courval et al, 1990). In the flaccid state, the muscles have abnormally low tone and volitional activity is lost. In the upper extremity, the force of gravity stretches the unsupported ligamentous structures near the glenohumeral joint. This may lead to shoulder subluxation and pain. If stretching of the joint capsule could be avoided during this acute and flaccid stage following a CVA, subsequent muscle return would reduce the incidence of chronic shoulder subluxation (Basmaijian and Bazant, 1986; Poulin de Courval et al, 1990; Van Ouwenaller et al, 1986). Reflex sympathetic dystrophy (RSD) is an autonomic nervous system disorder that often is the consequence of injury, immobilization, or both. It presents with changes in peripheral circulation, altered tolerance to movement and touch, chronic edema, loss of strength, and trophic changes of the skin and nails. Following a CVA, RSD is often called shoulder-hand dystrophy or shoulder-hand syndrome, and it may result in debilitating pain that is virtually impossible to eradicate (Falkenstein and Weiss-Lessard, 1999). The philosophy of treatment following a CVA is to incorporate regular movement of the joint within the pain-free range to thwart or prevent the onset of RSD and to use splinting only when needed for relief of muscle spasms or pain (Saidoff and McDonough, 1997; Tepperman et al, 1984). Unfortunately, the upper extremity of many post-CVA patients is placed in slings or supported on wheelchair lap trays or armrests. A sling that is incorrectly or inconsistently used does not prevent the stretching of the capsule or ligamentous support surrounding the glenohumeral joint. The sling adversely immobilizes the shoulder in adduction and internal rotation while encouraging a nonfunctional position of elbow and wrist flexion.

The use of electrical stimulation to the shoulder muscles may prevent overstretching of the glenohumeral capsule, thereby eliminating subluxation or the onset of RSD (Falkenstein and Weiss-Lessard, 1999; Saidoff and McDonald, 1997). Electrical stimulation, as an alternative to the shoulder sling, has been used since the 1980s (Baker et al, 1986). The current treatment regimen is electrical stimulation to the posterior deltoid and supraspinatus muscles (DeVahl, 1992). Electrical stimulation for up to 6 hours a day significantly reduces existing shoulder subluxation in the CVA patient and results in improved shoulder range of motion and electromyographic activity of the stimulated muscles (Faghri et al, 1994).

As flexion tone increases, patients are encouraged to perform self–range-of-motion exercises and functional activities with the affected upper extremity. A patient with moderate flexor spasticity tends to lose full extension of the wrist and fingers. Passive range-of-motion exercises can be coupled with electrical stimulation of the wrist and finger extensor muscles as an effective means of maintaining or increasing extension range of motion in the affected joints (Kraft et al, 1992; Baker et al, 1979). Electrical stimulation using two channels allows both the flexor and extensor muscles to be activated. In this case, the forearm is positioned on the ulnar surface, and the hand is rested on the fifth metacarpal to allow unrestricted flexion and extension. To increase joint motion in the presence of soft tissue contractures, passive stretching to the end range of motion and active movements should be accompanied by 4 hours of electrical stimulation each day (DeVahl, 1992).

Improvement in motor control following electrical stimulation at a current amplitude and frequency to produce muscle contraction has been well documented (Baker et al, 1979; Baker and Parker, 1986). In the post-CVA patient, it is important to pay attention to the duty cycle of the electrical stimulation. It has been determined that the 1:5 duty cycle ratio is the ideal setting for initial use in programs of prolonged stimulation of the wrist extensor or dorsiflexor muscles (Packman-Braun, 1988). The clinician, when using electrical stimulation on the patient with an injury to the nervous system, should carefully read the literature when deciding on the amount of time the electrical current is applied in relation to the amount of time allowed between onset of the stimulation period. Due to the confusion with parameters reported in published articles and quoted in vendor protocols, the reader is encouraged to decipher carefully from the methodology of the original research study the actual on-time and off-time for electrical stimulation. Finally, the term *duty cycle* is no longer preferred to describe the duration of current flow during a cycle of electrical stimulation. Reporting the actual on-time, off-time, and ramp times is the preferred method. See Chap. 1 for a description of the terminology for the duty cycle and on/off-times.

The use of electrical stimulation in conjunction with biofeedback electromyography (EMG) or a mirror has been shown to be a powerful adjunct to tactile and verbal cues for balance, posture, or muscle re-education (Bowman et al, 1979; Cozean et al, 1988; Kohlmeyer et al, 1996; Winchester et al, 1983).

The onset of electrical stimulation in each phase of the cycle is often delivered in a remote fashion using a pressure-sensitive switch either in the shoe of the patient (heel switch) or on a hand-held device controlled by the clinician. The remote switch is used in the acute phase of post-CVA rehabilitation to encourage postural alignment, dynamic sitting balance, or quadruped activities for the patient. The clinician can tap the remote switch positioned on the floor with his or her foot to activate delivery of electrical stimulation to the patient's trunk. This hands-free technique allows the clinician to provide balance support for the patient while ensuring that the onset of electrical stimulation coincides with a functional task and occurs in a temporal sequence meaningful to the patient's reacquisition of balance reactions.

The clinician can also the use the remote switch to assist the patient with grasp and release of an object, initiation or sequencing of movement, and sustaining contraction of a prime mover throughout the entire arc of movement. The hand-held switch may also be used to trigger stimulation of the dorsiflexor muscles during gait training. Alternatively, the clinician may control the onset of plantar flexor or hamstring muscle activity during the push-off or swing phase, respectively. This is in contrast to stimulation at the sole or dorsum of the foot to initiate the flexor reflex during the swing phase of gait with the spinal cord-injured patient (Cybulski et al, 1984).

Alternatively, the heel switch may also be placed in the patient's shoe to trigger the onset of stimulation (in the reverse mode) to the dorsiflexor muscles when weight is taken off the sensing device (Respond Select, EMPI, 599 Cardigan Rd, St. Paul, MN 55126). The dorsiflexors and foot evertor muscles are activated by stimulation of the peroneal nerve when the heel is lifted off of the pressure-sensitive heel switch. The parameters commonly used for electrical stimulation of the peroneal nerve include pulse durations from 20–250 µs, current amplitudes of less than 90 mA, and frequencies between 30–300 pps (Liberson et al, 1961). Alternatively, the electrode placement for dorsiflexion and eversion of the foot and ankle could include the motor points of the tibialis anterior and peroneal muscles. Electrical stimulation can also be applied to the gluteal or quadriceps muscles, or both during the stance phase of gait using the normal mode of stimulation triggered by weight-bearing on the heel switch. Thus, the sensing device in the heel switch could also be used to alternate stimulation between muscle groups using a dual channel arrangement.

Multichannel electrical stimulation is useful for rehabilitation following a CVA or head trauma when the patient has difficulty comprehending or following verbal instructions (Bogataj et al, 1995; Malezic et al, 1992; Stanic et al, 1978; Strojnik et al, 1979). After 1–3 weeks (5 days/week) of gait training with multichannel electrical stimulation at a 200 µs duration and 30 Hz frequency to the soleus, quadriceps, hamstring, gluteus maximus, triceps brachii muscles, and the peroneal nerve, measurable improvements in gait parameters were noted (Bogataj et al, 1989). Bogataj and associates enrolled 20 hemiplegic patients (4 head-injured and 16 CVA) in the study at 1.5–72 months postinjury. After 1–3 weeks of electrical stimulation, gait velocity increased an average of 61.6%, stride length increased an average of 46.3%, and the load transmitted from the affected leg to a force plate increased (Bogataj et al, 1989). Electrical stimulation to restore weight shift and symmetry of gait may include channels to stimulate the trunk extensor muscles, elevate the shoulder girdle, and initiate arm swing (Malezic et al, 1994). Malezic and colleagues reported that after 25 sessions with this multichannel system, 11 hemiplegic patients demonstrated an increase in gait velocity by 33%, stride length on the affected side by 26%, and a significant increase in weight shift to the affected side ($P = 0.05$).

PROCEDURE 11-1

Electrical Stimulation to Increase Range of Motion in the Upper Extremity of the Cerebrovascular Accident (CVA) or Head-injured Patient

Parameters	Settings
Current type/waveform	Pulsed current, square waveform
Pulse duration	200 μs
Current amplitude	As tolerated up to 100 mA, avoiding flexor withdrawal
Ramp up	3 seconds
Ramp down	None
Frequency	33 pps
On-time	7 seconds (includes ramp time)
Off-time	10 seconds
Treatment duration	15 minutes twice a day and then increased to 30 minutes three times a day and at night for 7 days/week for 4 weeks
Electrodes	Infant electrocardiogram electrodes with adhesive sponge backing
	New Dimensions in Medicine PO Box 1408 3040 E Rineir Rd Dayton, OH 45439
Electrode configuration	Cathode (–) over the motor points of the extensor carpi radialis longus (ECRL), extensor carpi radialis brevis (ECRB), extensor carpi ulnaris (ECU), and extensor digitorum (ED), just distal to the elbow; anode (+) was placed distally on the dorsal forearm near the wrist

(*continued*)

PROCEDURE 11–1

Continued

Parameters	Settings

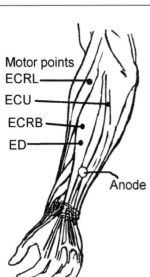

Motor points
ECRL
ECU
ECRB
ED

Anode

Electrical stimulation over the
motor points of the upper extremity to increase range of motion
after a cerebrovascular accident
(CVA) or head injury

Unit

Electrical Stimulation System
Neuromuscular Engineering
Department
Rancho Los Amigos Hospital
7601 E Imperial Hwy
Downey, CA 90242

OTHER: A positional splint was needed for some patients during electrical
stimulation to keep the metacarpal phalangeal (MP) joints in slight flexion in order to extend the proximal interphalangeal (PIP) and distal
interphalangeal (DIP) joints. In some patients, the wrist was positioned
in flexion to obtain greater extension force to overcome finger flexor
spasticity.

OUTCOME: Sixteen CVA or head-injured patients, 36–78 years of age,
were enrolled in the study at least 6 weeks postinjury. When severe
spasticity was present in the finger flexors, it was difficult to obtain
simultaneous extension of the wrist and fingers. Wrist and finger flexion

PROCEDURE 11–1

Continued

deformities were significantly reduced following 4 weeks of electrical stimulation ($P < 0.02$). When stimulation was discontinued, wrist extension range declined despite self–range-of-motion exercises. Those patients with active wrist extension prior to electrical stimulation demonstrated a slight increase in muscle mass.

SOURCE: Baker LL, Yeh C, Wilson D, Waters RL: Electrical stimulation of wrist and fingers for hemiplegic patients. *Phys Ther* 59(12):1495–1500, 1979.

PROCEDURE 11-2

Heel Switch Activated Electrical Stimulation During Gait Training of Hemiplegic Patients

Parameters	Settings
Current type/waveform	Monophasic pulsed current, rectangular waveform
Pulse duration	300 µs
Current amplitude	Up to 60 V
Frequency	25–50 Hz
On-time	4 seconds
Treatment duration	5 days/week × 7–21 days
Electrode configuration	Cathode (–), common peroneal nerve in the area between the popliteal fossa and the head of the fibula; anode (+), tibialis anterior

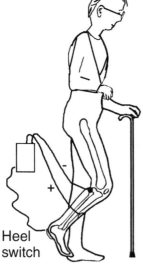

Heel switch

Heel switch-activated electrical stimulation of the peroneal nerve for correction of spastic foot drop in hemiplegia

OTHER: Heel switch activated dorsiflexion and inversion when the patient lifted his or her foot for a step. After 4 seconds, or when the heel hit the ground, the device reset automatically to discontinue stimulation.

PROCEDURE 11–2

Continued

OUTCOME: Nineteen hemiplegic patients (3–36 months post-CVA) were enrolled in the study. Significant improvement in inversion during initial stance ($P = 0.05$) on all surfaces and for symmetry of gait on linoleum was shown. Using the Barthel index to measure functional outcome, a significant improvement was noted when the electrical stimulation was used during gait ($P = 0.05$)

SOURCE: Granat MH, Maxwell DJ, Ferguson AC, et al: Peroneal stimulator: Evaluation for the correction of spastic drop foot in hemiplegia. *Arch Phys Med Rehabil* 77(1):19–24, 1996.

PROCEDURE 11–3

Electrical Stimulation for Muscle Reeducation of the Forearm and Hand in the Cerebrovascular Accident (CVA) Patient

Parameters	Settings
Current type	Symmetrical biphasic
Pulse duration	300 μs
Current amplitude	To desired response
Frequency	50 Hz
Treatment duration	Twice a day for 20–30 minutes × 24 weeks
Electrode configuration	Two channels for cathodes (–) are 4 × 3 karaya carbon rubber electrodes placed over the anterior and posterior forearm at least 2 cm proximal to the edge of the glove. The mesh-glove serves as the anode. Stimulation does not depend on particular positioning of the surface electrodes over the bellies of muscles or motor points

(–)
(–)
(+)

Glove anode for electrical stimulation of the hand in the hemiplegic patient

Unit	Respond II EMPI 599 Cardigan Rd St. Paul, MN 55126-3965

PROCEDURE **11–3**

Continued

Parameters	Settings
Mesh-glove*	Prizm-Medical, Inc. 4250 River Green Parkway Suite B Duluth GA 30136
	BioMedical Life-Systems 1120 Sycamore Ave Suite F Vista, CA 92083

OUTCOME: In the 1994 study, 40 post-CVA patients were enrolled and 14 post-CVA patients were enrolled in the 1996 study. Four protocols were used depending on the desired outcome: (1) control of spasticity, (2) awareness of hand and facilitation of movement, (3) conditioning of muscle disuse, or (4) relearning and augmentation of residual volitional movement. Following daily mesh-glove electrical stimulation, there was a significant improvement ($P < 0.05$) in wrist extension while coactivation of the biceps brachii decreased.

SOURCES:

Dimitrijević MM: Mesh-glove: 1. A method for whole-hand electrical stimulation in upper motor neuron dysfunction. *Scand J Rehab Med* 26(4):183–186, 1994.

Dimitrijević MM, Stokić DS, Wawro AW, Wun CC: Modification of motor control of wrist extension by mesh-glove electrical afferent stimulation in stroke patients. *Arch Phys Med Rehabil* 77(3):252–258, 1996.

* Mesh glove has been replaced by a line of Electro-mesh products including gloves, socks, and garment sleeves for elbow, knee, or limb electrical stimulation.

PROCEDURE 11–4

Electrical Stimulation to Prevent Shoulder Subluxation in Cerebrovascular Accident (CVA) Patients

Parameters	Settings
Current	Asymmetrical biphasic square wave
Pulse duration	300 µs
Current amplitude	30–35 mA, increased to 45 mA for a strong visible contraction without abduction or extension of the humerus
Ramp up	4 seconds
Ramp down	2 seconds
Frequency	30 pps
On-time	10 seconds
Off-time	20 seconds
Treatment duration	15 minutes two to four times daily, increased to 30 minutes after 1 week of stimulation, and then to 60 minute sessions
Electrode configuration	Supraspinatus and posterior deltoid for the first 2 weeks, then the middle or anterior deltoid instead of the posterior deltoid was stimulated

Electrode placement over the posterior deltoid and supraspinatus muscles for the prevention of shoulder subluxation

PROCEDURE 11–4

Continued

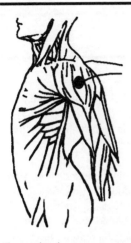

Electrode placement over the middle deltoid and supraspinatus muscles for the prevention of shoulder subluxation

Electrode placement over the anterior deltoid and supraspinatus muscles for the prevention of shoulder subluxation

OTHER: As the stimulation cycled on, the patient attempted to grasp objects of varying size and weight. The patient released the object as the stimulation cycled off.

OUTCOME: After 3 months, the patient was able to perform bilateral activities of daily living, dressing, and light housekeeping independently.

SOURCE: DeVahl J: Neuromuscular electrical stimulation (NMES) in rehabilitation, in *Electrotherapy in Rehabilitation*, MR Gersh (ed.). Philadelphia, FA Davis, 1992; pp 260–263.

PROCEDURE 11–5

Electrical Stimulation of the Flaccid Shoulder to Prevent Shoulder Subluxation in Cerebrovascular Accident (CVA) Patients

Parameters	Settings
Current type/waveform	Asymmetrical biphasic square wave
Current amplitude	High enough to produce humeral elevation with slight abduction and extension
Frequency	35 Hz
On-time	Progressively increased* from 10 to 12 seconds over 6 weeks
Off-time	Progressively decreased* from 30 to 2 seconds over 6 weeks
Treatment duration	Progressively increased from 1.5 to 6 hours/day, 7 days a week over 6 weeks
Electrode configuration	Cathode (–) over the posterior deltoid and the anode over the supraspinatus without stimulation of the trapezius

Electrode placement over the supraspinatus and posterior deltoid muscles for the prevention of shoulder subluxation

PROCEDURE 11–5

Continued

OTHER: Patients used wheelchair support trays or troughs whenever sitting.

OUTCOME: Twenty-six hemiplegic CVA patients with flaccid shoulder musculature were enrolled in the study at 17 ± 4 days post-CVA. The patients were divided into two groups that were matched for gender and affected side. One group received electrical stimulation, while the other served as the control. Patients were evaluated for arm muscle tone, function, EMG activity of the posterior deltoid muscle, subluxation (bilateral sitting radiographs), shoulder lateral range of motion, and pain. These evaluations occurred prior to electrical stimulation, after 6 weeks of electrical stimulation, and 6 weeks after completion of the study, and they revealed a significant difference in arm function, tone, and EMG activity between the two groups ($P < 0.05$). Radiographic analysis of the change in subluxation also demonstrated significant improvement for the group receiving 6 weeks of electrical stimulation when compared with the control group.

SOURCE: Faghri PD, Rodgers MM, Glaser RM, et al. The effects of functional electrical stimulation on shoulder subluxation, arm function recovery, and shoulder pain in hemiplegic stroke patients. *Arch Phys Med Rehabil* 75:73–79, 1994.

* When a patient was able to complete a 6 hour period of stimulation without muscle fatigue, progression of the on/off-time occurred. If the patient demonstrated no visible muscle response with maximal stimulation, progression of the on-/off-time did *not* occur.

PROCEDURE 11–6

Electrical Stimulation to Treat Shoulder Subluxation in Cerebrovascular Accident (CVA) Patients

Parameters	Settings
Current type/waveform	Asymmetrical biphasic pulsed current
Frequency	12–25 pps
On-time/Off-time	Increased from 1 : 3 to 12 : 1 (i.e. after a 6 week period, the on : off ratio was 24 seconds on : 2 seconds off)
Treatment duration	Initially, three 30 minute sessions, increased to 6–8 hours/day
Electrode configuration	Cathode (–) over posterior deltoid, anode (+) over supraspinatus

Electrode placement over the supraspinatus and posterior deltoid muscles for the prevention of shoulder subluxation

PROCEDURE 11-6

Continued

OUTCOME: After 6 weeks of electrical stimulation, radiographic analysis demonstrated an improvement in the glenohumeral position from an average distance of 14.8 mm to a distance of 8.6 mm. The control group, who did not receive electrical stimulation, did not show any significant improvement in the position of the humerus in the glenoid fossa.

SOURCE: Baker LL, Parker K: Neuromuscular electrical stimulation of the muscles surrounding the shoulder. *Phys Ther* 66:1930–1937, 1986.

References

Baker LL, Parker K: Neuromuscular electrical stimulation of the muscles surrounding the shoulder. *Phys Ther* 66:1930–1937, 1986.

Baker LL, Yeh C, Wilson D, Waters RL: Electrical stimulation of wrist and fingers for hemiplegic patients. *Phys Ther* 59(12):1495–1500, 1979.

Basmaijian JV, Bazant FJ: Factors preventing downward dislocation of the adducted shoulder joint: An electromyographic and morphological study. *JBJS* 41-A:1182–1186, 1986.

Bogataj U, Gros N, Kljajic M, et al: The rehabilitation of gait in patients with hemiplegia: A comparison between conventional therapy and multichannel functional electrical stimulation therapy. *Phys Ther* 75:490–502, 1995.

Bogataj U, Gros N, Malezic M, et al: Restoration of gait during two to three weeks of therapy with multichannel electrical stimulation. *Phys Ther* 69:319–327, 1989.

Bowman BR, Baker LL, Waters RL: Positional feedback and electrical stimulation: An automated treatment for the hemiplegic wrist. *Arch Phys Med Rehabil* 60:497–502, 1979.

Cozean C, Pease W, Hubbell S: Biofeedback and functional electrical stimulation in stroke rehabilitation. *Arch Phys Med Rehabil* 69:401–405, 1988.

Cybulski GR, Penn RD, Jaeger JF: Lower extremity functional neuromuscular stimulation in cases of spinal cord injury. *Neurosurg* 15:132–140, 1984.

DeVahl J: Neuromuscular electrical stimulation (NMES) in rehabilitation, in *Electrotherapy in Rehabilitation*, MR Gersh (ed.). Philadelphia, FA Davis, 1992; pp. 260–263.

Faghri PD, Rodgers MM, Glaser RM, et al: The effects of functional electrical stimulation on shoulder subluxation, arm function recovery, and shoulder pain in hemiplegic stroke patients. *Arch Phys Med Rehabil* 75:73–79, 1994.

Falkenstein N, Weiss-Lessard S: *Hand Rehabilitation: A Quick Reference Guide and Review*. St. Louis, Mosby, 1999; pp 143–151.

Kohlmeyer KM, Hill JP, Yarkony GM, Jaeger RJ: Electrical stimulation and biofeedback effect on recovery of tenodesis grasp: A controlled study. *Arch Phys Med Rehabil* 77:702–706, 1996.

Kraft GH, Fitts SS, Hammond MC: Techniques to improve function of the arm and hand in chronic hemiplegia. *Arch Phys Med Rehabil* 73:220–227, 1992.

Liberson WT, Holmquist HJ, Scott D, Dow M: Functional electrotherapy: Stimulation of the peroneal nerve synchronized with the swing phase of gait of hemiplegic patients. *Arch Phys Med Rehabil* 42:101–105, 1961.

Malezic M, Bogataj U, Gros N, et al: Application of a programmable dual-channel adaptive electrical stimulation system for the control and analysis of gait. *J Rehabil Res Dev* 29(4):41–53, 1992.

Malezic M, Hesse S, Schewe H, et al: Restoration of standing, weight-shift and gait by multichannel electrical stimulation in hemiparetic patients. *Int J Rehabil Res* 17(2):169–179, 1994.

Packman-Braun R: Relationship between functional electrical stimulation duty cycle and fatigue in wrist extensor muscles of patients with hemiparesis. *Phys Ther* 68(1):51–56, 1988.

Poulin de Courval L, Barsauskas A, Berenbaum B, et al: Painful shoulder in the hemiplegic and unilateral neglect. *Arch Phys Med Rehabil* 71:673–676, 1990.

Saidoff DC, McDonough AL: *Critical Pathways in Therapeutic Intervention: Upper Extremity.* St. Louis, Mosby, 1997; pp 52–65.

Stanic U, Acimovic-Janezic R, Gros N, et al: Multichannel electrical stimulation for correction of hemiplegic gait. Methodology and Preliminary Results. *Scand J Rehabil Med* 10(2):75–92, 1978.

Strojnik P, Kralj A, Ursic I: Programmed six-channel electrical stimulator for complex stimulation of leg muscles during walking. *IEE Trans Biomed Eng* 26(2):112–116, 1979.

Tepperman PS, Greyson ND, Hilbert L, et al: Reflex sympathetic dystrophy in hemiplegia. *Arch Phys Med Rehabil* 65:442–447, 1984.

Van Ouwenaller C, LaPlace PM, Chantraine A: Painful shoulder in hemiplegia. *Arch Phys Med Rehabil* 67:23–26, 1986.

Winchester P, Montgomery J, Bowman B, Hislop H: Effects of feedback stimulation training and cyclical electrical stimulation on knee extension in hemiparetic patients. *Phys Ther* 63:1096–1103, 1983.

.

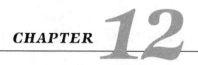

Pediatric Electrotherapy

Electrical stimulation of the developing nervous system of a child has not been extensively researched; however, there are several reports in the literature of the effectiveness of electrical stimulation for children with cerebral palsy, Duchenne's muscular dystrophy (DMD), spina bifida, scoliosis, and other disorders. It is important to realize that the values for electrical stimulation used on the adolescent or adult *cannot* be used on the child under 5 years of age due to the ongoing myelination process.

Myelination of the peripheral nerves occurs at different rates. For example, the ulnar motor responses may mature faster than the median nerve responses within the same limb. Similarly, until 5 years of age, peroneal motor responses may mature faster than tibial nerve responses (Stempien, 1998).

The motor nerve conduction velocities are only 19 meters/second in premature infants, 20–30 meters/second in full term newborn infants, and do not reach adult values until 4–5 years of age (Wagner and Buchtal, 1972). Due to the immature neuromuscular junction, stimulation frequencies greater than 20 pps or 20 Hz result in a decremental response of the compound muscle action potential (Cornblath, 1986; Navarette and Vrbová, 1983). In children less than 3 years of age, the motor units are immature, resulting in an inconsistent recruitment pattern (Sacco et al, 1962).

Injury to the nerve in a child may be the result of a fracture, thoracic surgery, or obstetric brachial plexus palsy. Mononeuropathy may be the result of repetitive activity, such as wheelchair propulsion. Overuse of the fingers in repetitive motions, such as are needed to use the keyboard, mouse, or electronic game controller, is becoming more common in children. Entrapment of the nerve may occur at the elbow and wrist. Traumatic injuries occur frequently to the distal radial nerve trunk and the posterior interosseous nerve (Stempien, 1998). Compression of the peroneal nerve occurs frequently in children (Jones et al, 1993). In all of these cases, there is a very optimistic prognosis for recovery of function with at least 75% of the children showing significant improvement (Stempien, 1998).

It is important for the clinician to remember that peripheral nerves may be affected by systemic diseases, such as mucolipidosis and scleroderma, or from tumors, such as osteoid osteoma or lymphoma. Hereditary sensory motor neuropathies (including Charcot-Marie-Tooth disease), acute inflammatory demyelinating polyneuropathy (Guillain-Barre syndrome), spinal muscular atrophy, human immunodeficiency virus (HIV), lead poisoning, botulism, tick bites, insect or snake venom, organophosphate exposure, adverse reaction to antibiotics or chemotherapy, metabolic disorders, and vasculitis can adversely affect motor nerve conduction velocity and the compound muscle action potential (Jones et al, 1996; Ouvrier et al, 1990; Stempien, 1998).

In the case of neuromuscular disease, electrical stimulation delivers an activity pattern to the skeletal muscle that is beneficial, whether the motor neuron is directly involved or not (Pette and Vrbová 1985; Scott et al, 1986). In the case of DMD, there is slow contraction and relaxation of the muscles, so it is important to use only a low frequency of electrical stimulation (less than 30 pps), similar to that used in the immature nervous system (Dubowitz et al, 1987). Hypertrophy of the dystrophic muscle, an undesirable effect of DMD, is unlikely at low frequency electrical stimulation, due to a low ratio of muscle fiber recruitment. Chronic electrical stimulation for 250 ms every second for 4 minutes does not result in muscle fatigue or loss of force in the child with DMD (Scott et al, 1986).

Children as old as 16 years of age with cerebral palsy demonstrate muscle property changes adversely affecting gait (Berger et al, 1982). Therapeutic electrical stimulation (TES) uses low level stimulation

(<10 mA) applied during sleep for 8–12 hours with resultant increases in muscle bulk within 6–8 weeks. In conjunction with strengthening exercises and functional retraining, improved functional levels are noted within 6–12 months of nightly electrical stimulation (Pape, 1993; Pape et al, 1997).

Orthopedic or postoperative application of electrical stimulation to the child while the leg is immobilized in a short leg cast has been described. Markers are placed at the electrode sites prior to the application of the cast. After the cast has dried, windows are cut in the cast to expose the marker sites. Once the electrodes are in place, the cast windows are closed and secured with tape or an ace wrap (DeVahl, 1992).

Introducing electrical stimulation to the child may require several preliminary sessions without the use of current. The recommended guidelines follow.

1. Accommodate the child to the sensation of a hand-held vibrator or vibrating toy (Minimassager, Smith & Nephew Rolyan, Inc, PO Box 1005, Germantown, WI 53022). Begin by allowing time for the child to listen to the sounds before briefly (1–2 seconds) touching the child's thigh (if sensate). Do not begin at the child's hand, due to the high concentration of sensory nerve endings. Progress only as tolerated by the child. Involve the child in the "game" by letting him or her position the vibrating device.

2. Show the child the electrical stimulator and the electrodes. Let the child touch the sticky surface of the electrode. Apply the electrodes in the desired positions but do not turn on the amplitude. Attach the electrode wires.

3. At the next session explain to the child that he or she will feel a vibrating or tapping sensation under the electrode. Lightly tap the electrode to illustrate the sensation. If the child appears fearful, repeat step 1.

4. With the electrodes applied in the appropriate position, adjust the frequency to no more than 10 pps. The stimulation amplitude should be only at a sensory level until the child is comfortable with the procedure. Observe the child's facial expressions, breathing pattern, and heart rate. Sensory stimulation may be all that is tolerated by the child during this session.

5. To proceed to motor stimulation, increase the frequency but do not exceed 20 pps if the child is under 5 years of age. The ampli-

tude should not be increased beyond a level producing a tingling sensation.

6. The electrodes should not be smaller than 2 cm. If trimming the electrodes, take care not to disrupt the internal lead embedded within the electrode surface.
7. If overflow to the antagonist muscle occurs, move the inactive electrode closer to the active electrode to create a superficial current flow.
8. Do not treat longer than 10 minutes for the first several sessions.
9. Monitor skin reaction carefully immediately after the session and through parental reports of the skin appearance for hours after the treatment.

PROCEDURE 12–1

Electrical Stimulation of the Ankle of a Hemiplegic Cerebral Palsied Child

Parameters	Settings
Current type/waveform	Asymmetrical biphasic pulsed current
Pulse duration	300 μs
Current amplitude	Increase very slowly, but never to maximal contraction
Ramp up	8 seconds for motor retraining *or* 0.5 seconds for gait training
Ramp down	8 seconds for motor retraining *or* 0.5 seconds for gait training
Frequency	5–7 pps and increased gradually to 30–35 pps
On-time	10 seconds*
Off-time	25 seconds*
Treatment duration	15–20 minutes
Electrode configuration	Pregelled, self-adhering, reusable carbon electrodes placed with the active electrode on the motor point and the inactive electrode on the same muscle group. Electrodes are cut to fit the child's extremity but are never smaller than an inch in diameter. Some children may require alternating stimulation of the dorsiflexors and plantar flexors during gait

Electrical stimulation to enhance motor control of the dorsiflexor muscles and improve balance in the hemiplegic cerebral palsied child

(*continued*)

* Once the child is comfortable with electrical stimulation and not showing signs of fatigue, the cycle can be set to 15 seconds on and 15 seconds off.

PROCEDURE 12–1

Continued

Parameters	Settings
Unit/company	Respond II EMPI 599 Cardigan Rd St. Paul, MN 55126 (Formerly of Medtronic)

OUTCOME: Three children (ages 1, 6, and 10 years) demonstrated improvements in balance and motor control of the dorsiflexor muscles. Gait results were varied, warranting further study with a larger sample size.

SOURCE: Carmick J: Clinical use of neuromuscular electrical stimulation for children with cerebral palsy. Part I: Lower extremity. *Phys Ther* 73(8):505–513, 1993.

PROCEDURE 12–2

Electrical Stimulation of the Hemiplegic Cerebral Palsied Child's Wrist

Parameters	Settings
Current type/waveform	Asymmetrical biphasic pulsed current
Pulse duration	300 μs
Current amplitude	Increased very slowly but never to maximal contraction
Ramp up	8 seconds for motor retraining, 0.5 seconds for faster movements
Ramp down	8 seconds for motor retraining
Frequency	5–7 pps and increased gradually to 30–35 pps
On-time	10 seconds*
Off-time	25 seconds*
Treatment duration	15–20 minutes
Electrode configuration	Active electrode is placed on the motor point, and the inactive electrode is placed on the same muscle group. Electrodes are cut to fit the child's extremity but are never smaller than an inch in diameter

Electrical stimulation of the wrist extensors to improve function in the hemiplegic cerebral palsied child

(*continued*)

* Once the child is comfortable with electrical stimulation and not showing signs of fatigue, the cycle can be set to 15 seconds on and 15 seconds off.

PROCEDURE 12–2

Continued

Parameters	Settings
Remote switch	Activates wrist extensors when child picks up an object. Finger extensors activated to allow the child to release object. No current flows to electrodes when the child moves arm to pick up another object
Unit/company	Respond II EMPI 599 Cardigan Rd St. Paul, MN 55126 (Formerly of Medtronic)
Pedi electrodes/company	Uni-Patch Encore Plus Electrodes Uni-Patch, Inc 1313 Grand Blvd West PO Box 271 Wabasha, MN 55981

OUTCOME: Case study with two children (ages 1 and 6 years) describing improvements in functional and sensory awareness.

SOURCE: Carmick J: Clinical use of neuromuscular electrical stimulation for children with cerebral palsy. Part 2: Upper extremity. *Phys Ther* 73(8):514–522, 1993.

PROCEDURE 12–3

Electrical Stimulation of the Wrist in Conjunction with a Dorsal Wrist Splint for a Hemiplegic Cerebral Palsied Child

Parameters	Settings
Current type/waveform	Asymmetrical biphasic pulsed current
Pulse duration	300 μs
Current amplitude	Increase very slowly but never to maximal contraction
Ramp up	0.5 seconds
Frequency	35 pps
On-time	15 seconds (when remote switch is not used)
Off-time	15 seconds (when remote switch is not used)
Remote trigger	Alternating mode so that finger flexion was facilitated when the remote switch is depressed and finger extension is facilitated when the switch was released
Treatment duration	15–20 minutes weekly
Electrode configuration	*Wrist flexion* Active: motor point Inactive: near wrist *Wrist extension* Active: near elbow Inactive: near wrist *Finger extension* Active: between elbow and wrist Inactive: near wrist *Finger flexors* Active: between wrist and cubital fossa Inactive: near wrist

Enhancement of wrist and hand function in the child with cerebral palsy

(continued)

PROCEDURE 12–3

Continued

Parameters	Settings
	The inactive electrode for the wrist and finger extensors was shared. Both electrodes on the anterior forearm were connected to channel one
In conjunction with dorsal wrist splint	Orthoplast (Johnson & Johnson Orthopaedics) custom splint used for sensory stimulation of the extensor surface. Wrist positioned in 10° extension with anchor at distal ulna. Dorsal wrist splint covered the forearm and dorsal hand up to the metacarpal phalangeal (MP) joints. Splint is designed to prevent ulnar deviation or excessive wrist extension with two forearm straps and one soft palmar strap/web space strap. Electrodes used under splint
Unit/company	Respond and Respond II dual channel with remote trigger EMPI 599 Cardigan Rd St. Paul, MN 55126 (800) 328-2536
Electrodes/company	Uni-Patch Encore Plus Electrodes Uni-Patch, Inc 1313 Grand Blvd West PO Box 271 Wabasha, MN 55981

OUTCOME: The dorsal wrist splint improved hand function after 24 sessions of wearing the splint at least 6 hours/day.

SOURCE: Carmick J: Use of neuromuscular electrical stimulation and a dorsal wrist splint to improve the hand function of a child with spastic hemiparesis. *Phys Ther* 77(6):661–671, 1997.

PROCEDURE 12–4

Electrical Stimulation of the Child
With Hemiplegic Cerebral Palsy

Parameters	Settings
Current type/waveform	Asymmetrical biphasic pulsed current
Pulse duration	Gradually increase over a week to 100 μs
Current amplitude	Gradually increase over a week to provide a range of dorsiflexion slightly less than the individual's passive range of motion
Ramp up	2 seconds (included in the on-time)
Frequency	30 pps
On-time	7 seconds
Off-time	15 seconds
Treatment duration	1 hour/day for 5 weeks
Electrode configuration	Self-adhering on the motor points of the tibialis anterior and extensor digitorum

Electrical stimulation of the tibialis anterior and extensor digitorum muscles in the child with
cerebral palsy

Unit/company	In Britain: DMI stimulator DMI Medical Ltd. Wigan, England

OTHER: Children could perform any functional activity desired while
receiving the electrical stimulation.

(continued)

PROCEDURE 12–4

Continued

OUTCOME: Twenty hemiplegic cerebral palsied children, 5 to 12 years of age, were enrolled in the study. The children were age-matched with 80% matched within a year of age. One of each pair received electrical stimulation, while the other child in the pair served as the control. After 35 consecutive days of electrical stimulation to the tibialis anterior and extensor digitorum, there was a significant increase in ankle dorsiflexion with the knee extended ($P = 0.05$). There was a statistically significant difference in the active voluntary dorsiflexion in sitting when comparing the control and treatment groups ($P = 0.03$), but there was not a significant change in the pretest and posttest measurements in either the control or treatment groups for this same variable. There was, however, a significant improvement in the strength of the tibialis anterior muscle when comparing the pretest and posttest of the electrically stimulated group ($P = 0.02$). The authors did not comment on change in muscle tone but addressed the difficulty in determining the strength in the presence of abnormal tone. There was no apprehension from the children about the use of electrical stimulation. There were no adverse reactions from applying electrical stimulation across a joint with a contracture since the joint was allowed to move below the limit of the available range of motion. A twin axis electrogoniometer with visual angle display was used to measure rotational displacement of one limb segment relative to the other, irrespective of the axis of the joint.

SOURCE: Hazlewood ME, Brown JK, Rowe PJ, Salter PM: The use of therapeutic electrical stimulation in the treatment of hemiplegic cerebral palsy. *Dev Med Child Neurol* 36:661–673, 1994.

PROCEDURE 12–5

Electrical Stimulation of the Child With Diplegic or Hemiplegic Cerebral Palsy

Parameters	Settings
Current type/waveform	Biphasic pulsed current
Pulse duration	300 μs
Current amplitude	< 10 mA
Ramp up	2 seconds
Frequency	35–45 pps
On/off-time	1 : 1
Treatment duration	An average of 9 hours/night during sleep
Electrode configuration	1 × 2 inch silicone rubber electrodes to the tibialis anterior muscle for a 6 month period, followed by a 6 month period without electrical stimulation. Another 6 month period of electrical stimulation was then repeated; however, the quadriceps muscle group was stimulated in addition to the tibialis anterior muscle

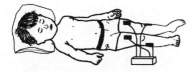

Electrical stimulation of the hemiplegic or diplegic cerebral palsied child to enhance gait, balance, and gross motor function

OUTCOME: Six ambulatory children (3–6 years of age) with mild spastic diplegia or hemiplegia were patients in this single-subject study. Of the five children who completed 6 months of electrical stimulation to the tibialis anterior muscle, there was significant improvement in function as quantified with the Peabody Developmental Motor Scales. After 6 months of no electrical stimulation, the scores for each of the five skill sections of the Peabody fell back toward the baseline level. When electrical stimulation was reinstated to include the tibialis anterior and the quadriceps muscles, the Peabody scores improved and were once again significantly different than the baseline findings taken 1.5 years previously at the beginning of the study. Three of the skill levels (total gross motor, balance, and locomotor) were significantly

(continued)

PROCEDURE 12–5

Continued

betted after the second 6 month period of electrical stimulation than
reported following the first 6 month period of electrical stimulation
indicating that the 6 month "off" period was not detrimental to the
overall success of the treatment. The authors ruled out the possibility
of spontaneous recovery of function and attributed the findings to
differential growth of nonspastic antagonist muscle during electrical
stimulation while sleeping.

SOURCE: Pape KE, Kirsch SE, Galil A, et al: Neuromuscular approach to the motor deficits of
cerebral palsy: A pilot study. *J Pediatr Orthop* 13(5):628–633, 1993.

PROCEDURE 12–6

Electrical Stimulation During the Gait of the Child with Diplegic or Hemiplegic Cerebral Palsy

Introduction of Electrical Stimulation Sensation to the Child

Duration is 1–2 sessions.

Parameters	Settings
Current type/waveform	Biphasic pulsed current
Current amplitude	To tapping sensory level for several minutes followed by visible motor response
Ramp up	5–10 seconds
Frequency	5–10 pps
On-time	10 seconds (does not include ramp times)
Off-time	25 seconds
Treatment duration	15 minutes

Gait Settings

Parameters	Settings
Current type/waveform	Biphasic pulsed current
Current amplitude	Visible motor response
Ramp up	0.5 seconds
Frequency	32 pps
Treatment duration	Phase one: 15 minutes, three times weekly × 4 weeks
	Phase two: 15 minutes, three times weekly × 4 weeks
Electrode configuration	Phase one: Active electrode on the motor point of the gastrocnemius, and the inactive electrode on the same muscle a short distance away
	Phase two:
	Channel One: Active electrode on the motor point of the gastrocnemius, and the inactive electrode on the same muscle a short distance away

(continued)

PROCEDURE 12–6

Continued

Parameters	Settings
	Channel Two: Active electrode on the motor point of the tibialis anterior, and the inactive electrode on the same muscle a short distance away
Remote switch	*Phase one:* The current flow to the gastrocnemius was allowed to flow just before heel strike and released just after toe-off using a remote switch controlled by the investigator
	Phase two: Reciprocal mode so that current flows only to channel one to activate gastrocnemius when the switch was depressed, and then only to channel two to activate the tibialis anterior when the switch was released
Unit/company	Respond II Select EMPI 599 Cardigan Rd St. Paul, MN 55126 (800) 328-2536 (Formerly of Medtronic.)

OUTCOME: Four children with hemiplegic cerebral palsy and ten children with diplegic cerebral palsy between the ages of 4 and 14 years were enrolled in the study. All were independent ambulators, but all lacked heel strike. There was a significant difference in ankle dorsiflexion at initial foot contact during gait with either electrical stimulation of the gastrocnemius or reciprocal stimulation of the gastrocnemius and tibialis anterior muscles.

SOURCE: Comeaux P, Patterson N, Rubin M, Meiner R: Effect of neuromuscular electrical stimulation during gait in children with cerebral palsy. *Pediatr Phys Ther* 9:103–109, 1997.

PROCEDURE 12–7

Electrical Stimulation of the Child
With Spina Bifida

Parameters	Settings
Current type/waveform	Biphasic pulsed current, rectangular waveform
Pulse duration	347 μs
Current amplitude	50 mA
Ramp up	2 seconds
Ramp down	5 seconds
Frequency	35 pps
On-time week 1	8 seconds (excluding ramp time)
Off-time week 1	24 seconds
On-time week 2	8 seconds (excluding ramp time)
Off-time week 2	16 seconds
On-time weeks 3 through 8	8 seconds
Off-time weeks 3 through 8	8 seconds (excluding ramp time)
Treatment duration	30 min/day, 6 d /wk, × 8 weeks
Electrode configuration	Pregelled electrode (4.4 × 8.9 cm) over the vastus lateralis and rectus femoris; second electrode over rectus femoris and vastus medialis

Electrical stimulation to enhance upright function of the child with spina bifida

(continued)

PROCEDURE 12-7
Continued

Parameters	Settings
Exercise in conjunction with stimulation	Stand or move in an upright position while using regular orthosis
Unit/company	Myocare neuromuscular stimulator Medical-Surgical Division 3M 3M Center St. Paul, MN 55144

OUTCOME: Two children 5 years of age, two children 12 years of age, and one 21-year-old adult were enrolled in the study. By week 8, the stimulated limb of one of the 12-year-old children became stronger than the contralateral control limb at 45° and 60° knee extension. There was, however, no significant difference between the peak torque measurements of either the electrically stimulated limb or the contralateral control limb at any angle of extension. The 12-year-olds ascended 20 stairs or descended 20 stairs at a rate of 0–3 seconds faster after 8 weeks of electrical stimulation to the quadriceps muscle. Three out of four of the children 5–12 years of age improved their time in walking 80 feet over a level surface by 3–5 seconds after 8 weeks of electrical stimulation.

SOURCE: Karmel-Ross K, Cooperman DR, Van Doren CL: The effect of electrical stimulation on quadriceps femoris muscle torque in children with spina bifida. *Phys Ther* 72(10):723–730, 1992.

PROCEDURE 12-8

Electrical Stimulation of Children With Duchenne Muscular Dystrophy (DMD)

Parameters	Settings
Current type/waveform	Biphasic pulsed current
Pulse duration	50 μs
Frequency	5–10 pps
On-time	1–5 seconds
Off-time	1–5 seconds
Treatment duration	1 hour three times daily for 7–11 weeks
Electrode configuration	Two 4 cm carbon electrodes on the tibialis anterior muscle

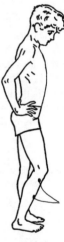

Electrical stimulation of the tibialis anterior to enhance functional gait in the child with Duchenne muscular dystrophy (DMD)

OUTCOME: Sixteen boys, 5–12 years of age, were enrolled in the study. Of these, 12 were independent ambulators, two required assistance to walk, and two were wheelchair-bound. In six of the ambulatory children, there was a significant increase ($P < 0.05$) in the mean maximum voluntary contraction compared with the contralateral limb, which did not receive electrical stimulation. The muscles of children with DMD demonstrated fatigue resistance to chronic low frequency electrical stimulation.

SOURCE: Scott OM, Vrbová G, Hyde SA, Dubowitz V: Responses of muscles of patients with Duchenne muscular dystrophy to chronic electrical stimulation. J Neurol Neurosurg Psychiatr 49:1427–1434, 1986.

PROCEDURE 12–9

Electrical Stimulation on Children With Duchenne Muscular Dystrophy (DMD)

Parameters	Settings
Current type/waveform	Biphasic asymmetrical current
Cycle duration	290 μs
Current amplitude	50 mA
Frequency	8 Hz
On-time	1.5 seconds
Off-time	1.5 seconds
Treatment duration	3 hours/day, 6 days/week for 10–11 weeks
Electrode configuration	Two carbon electrodes (4 × 9.5 cm)

OUTCOME: The maximum voluntary contraction of the quadriceps muscle of 34 healthy children, 4–13 years of age, was compared with that of 15 boys, 4–13 years of age with DMD. None of the boys had hip or knee contractures greater than 5°, but two boys had equinus contractures greater than 20° prior to the initiation of electrical stimulation. After 10 weeks of electrical stimulation, all 15 boys with DMD demonstrated a significant increase in the maximum voluntary contraction of the stimulated muscle ($P < 0.01$).

SOURCE: Scott OM, Hyde SA, Vrbová G, Dubowitz V: Therapeutic possibilities of chronic low frequency electrical stimulation in children with Duchenne muscular dystrophy. J Neurol Sci 95:171–182, 1990.

PROCEDURE 12–10

Electrical Stimulation of 3-Year-Old Children Who Were Born Premature With Resultant Intraventricular Hemorrhage and Hemiplegic Cerebral Palsy

Parameters	Settings
Current type/waveform	Biphasic pulsed current, square waveform
Pulse duration	20 μs
Frequency	5–10 pps
On-time	1–5 seconds
Off-time	1–5 seconds
Treatment duration	1 hour, three times daily for 8 weeks
Electrode configuration	Two 4 cm² carbon electrodes on the tibialis anterior muscle: one on the motor point, the other on the muscle belly

Electrical stimulation of the hemiplegic 3-year-old child

OUTCOME: Two girls born premature with resultant intraventricular hemorrhage with parenchymal extension and a porencephalic cyst were described in this case report. One child received a ventriculoperitoneal shunt at 8 weeks of age, but at 18 months still demonstrated an enlarged ventricle, cortical atrophy, and delayed myelination on the right side of the brain. At the initiation of the study, this child presented with left

(continued)

PROCEDURE 12–10

Continued

___

hemiplegia and no active dorsiflexion. In addition, there was a dominance of the flexion synergy pattern in the lower extremity. After 8 weeks of electrical stimulation, active dorsiflexion was possible. Isolated joint movements on the left lower extremity were possible with the emergence of equilibrium reactions. The second child underwent bilateral ventricular taps, but at 3 years of age demonstrated persistent ventriculomegaly and bilateral delayed myelination (left > right, posterior > anterior). Clinically, this child presented with right hemiplegia with weak active dorsiflexion prior to electrical stimulation. After 8 weeks of electrical stimulation, she demonstrated improvement in static and dynamic standing balance.

___

SOURCE: Dubowitz L, Finnie N, Hyde SA, et al: Improvement of muscle performance by chronic electrical stimulation in children with cerebral palsy. *Lancet* 1:587–588, 1988.

PROCEDURE 12–11

Lateral Electrical Stimulation for the Treatment of Scoliosis

Parameters	Settings
Current type/waveform	Symmetrical biphasic
Cycle duration	150 μs
Mode	Surged
Current amplitude	Slightly above motor threshold
Frequency	80–100 Hz
On-time	3 seconds
Off-time	3 seconds
Treatment duration	8 hours while sleeping
Electrode configuration	Both electrodes on the convexity of the curve

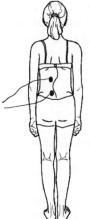

Electrical stimulation while sleeping to control the progression of scoliosis

OTHER: Patients who are considered candidates for this procedure must have curves measuring 29–45° by the Cobb method and have at least 1 year of spinal growth remaining.

SOURCE: Kahn J: *Principles and Practice of Electrotherapy,* 3d ed. New York, Churchill Livingstone, 1994; p 104.

PROCEDURE 12–12

Electrical Stimulation at Night in Conjunction With Bracing During the Day for Adolescents With Scoliosis

Parameters	Settings
Current type/waveform	Monophasic continuous current, rectangular waveform
Pulse duration	200 μs
Current amplitude	60–80 mA
Frequency	25 pps
On-time	6 seconds
Off-time	6 seconds
Treatment duration	8 hours at night
Electrode configuration	Two electrodes: one above and one below the apex of the curve at a distance between 6 and 16 cm apart

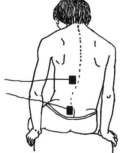

Nighttime electrical stimulation for use with daytime bracing in the adolescent with scoliosis

OTHER: Patients who are considered candidates for this procedure must have curves measuring 29–45° by the Cobb method and have at least 1 year of spinal growth remaining. This method has not been shown to be beneficial over bracing and should *not* be used in lieu of bracing.

SOURCES:

Francis EE: Lateral electrical surface stimulation treatment for scoliosis. *Pediatric Nursing* 13(3):157–160, 1987.

Sullivan J, Davidson R, Renshaw T, et al: Further evaluation of the Scolitron treatment of idiopathic adolescent scoliosis. *Spine* 11(2):903–906, 1986.

PROCEDURE 12–13

Lateral Electrical Stimulation for the Treatment of Thoracic Scoliosis

Parameters	Settings
Current type/waveform	Monophasic pulsed current, rectangular waveform
Pulse duration	220 µs
Current amplitude	Gradually increased until muscle contraction is strong
Frequency	25 pps
On-time	6 seconds
Off-time	6 seconds
Treatment duration	Gradually increase to 8 hours while sleeping; used each night until skeletal maturity
Electrode configuration	Midaxillary line on the convex side of the curve. One electrode is placed slightly above the rib that is attached to the apical vertebra, and the other electrode is placed slightly below the rib that is attached to the apical vertebra. If a double major or compensatory curve exists, a second channel is used with electrode placement on the convex side of the curve around the apical vertebra

Electrode placement for midaxillary electrical stimulation of a double major scoliotic curve

(continued)

PROCEDURE 12–13

Continued

OTHER: Patients who are considered candidates for this procedure must have curves measuring 29–45° by the Cobb method and have at least 1 year of spinal growth remaining.

OUTCOME: There was an 82% compliance, with 72% of the patients demonstrating a reduction or halt in the curve progression.

SOURCES:

Axelgaard J, Brown JC: Lateral electrical surface stimulation for the treatment of progressive idiopathic scoliosis. *Spine* 8:242–260, 1983.

Brown JC, Axelgaard J, Howson DC: Multicenter trial of a noninvasive stimulation method for idiopathic scoliosis. *Spine* 9:382–387, 1984.

Eckerson LF, Axelgaard J: Lateral electrical surface stimulation as an alternative to bracing in the treatment of idiopathic scoliosis. *Phys Ther* 64:483–490, 1984.

PROCEDURE 12–14

Electrical Stimulation for the Treatment of Idiopathic Scoliosis

Parameters	Settings
Current type/waveform	Biphasic pulsed current
Pulse duration	200 μs
Mode	Surged
Current amplitude	5–100 mA
Frequency	35 pps
On-time	5 seconds
Off-time	25 seconds
Treatment duration	8–10 hours while sleeping
Electrode configuration	Both electrodes on the convexity of the curve 1–3 inches lateral to the spine, with one electrode 3 inches above the apex and the other electrode 3 inches below the apex of the curve

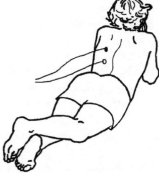

Electrical stimulation while sleeping in patients with scoliotic curves less than 40° and with 2 years of skeletal growth remaining

OTHER: Patients who are considered candidates for this procedure must have curves measuring less than 45° by the Cobb method and have at least 2 years of spinal growth remaining.

OUTCOME: Fisher and coworkers reported that there was no significant difference between electrical stimulation and bracing in the treatment of scoliotic curves (20–40°) in adolescents. Following a multicenter study with 379 patients, McCollough reported that electrical stimulation halted curve progression in over 90% of the patients with curves less than 30°.

SOURCES:

Fisher DA, Rapp GF, Emkes M: Idiopathic scoliosis: Transcutaneous muscle stimulation versus the Milwaukee brace. *Spine* 12:987–991, 1987.

McCollough NC: Nonoperative treatment of idiopathic scoliosis using surface electrical stimulation. *Spine* 11:802–804, 1986.

References

Berger W, Quinlun J, Dietz V: Pathophysiology of gait in children with cerebral palsy. *Electroencephel Clin Neurophysiol* 53:538–548, 1982.

Cornblath DR: Disorders of neuromuscular transmission in infants and children. *Muscle Nerve* 9:606–611, 1986.

DeVahl J: Neuromuscular electrical stimulation (NMES) in rehabilitation, in MR Gersh, *Electrotherapy in Rehabilitation*. Philadelphia, FA Davis, 1992; p 256.

Dubowitz V, Hyde SA, Scott OM, Vrbová G: Effects of chronic high frequency stimulation on muscles of children with Duchenne muscular dystrophy. *J Physiol* 390:132, 1987.

Jones HR, Bolton CF, Harper CM: *Pediatric Clinical Electromyography*. Philadelphia, Lippincott-Raven, 1996.

Jones HR Jr, Felice KJ, Gross PT: Pediatric peroneal mononeuropathy: A clinical and electromyographic study. *Muscle Nerve* 16:1167–1173, 1993.

Navarette R, Vrbová G: Changes of activity patterns in slow and fast muscles during postnatal development. *Develop Brain Res* 8:11–19, 1983.

Ouvrier RA, McLeod JG, Pollard JD: *Peripheral Neuropathy in Childhood*. New York, Raven, 1990.

Pape KE: Therapeutic electrical stimulation (TES) for the treatment of disuse muscle atrophy in cerebral palsy. *Pediatr Phys Ther* 9:110–112, 1997.

Pape KE, Kirsch SE, Galil A, et al: Neuromuscular approach to the motor deficits of cerebral palsy: A pilot study. *J Pediatr Orthop* 13(5):628–633, 1993.

Pette D, Vrbová G: Control of the phenotype expression in mammalian muscle fibres. *Muscle Nerve* 8:676–689, 1985.

Sacco G, Buchthal F, Rosenfalek P: Motor unit potentials at different ages. *Arch Neurol* 6:366–373, 1962.

Scott OM, Hyde SA, Vrbová G, Dubowitz V: Therapeutic possibilities of chronic low frequency electrical stimulation in children with Duchenne muscular dystrophy. *J Neurol Sci* 95:171–182, 1990.

Scott OM, Vrbová G, Hyde SA, Dubowitz V: Responses of muscles of patients with Duchenne muscular dystrophy to chronic electrical stimulation. *J Neurol Neurosurg Psychiatr* 49:1427–1434, 1986.

Stempien LM: Special considerations in pediatric electromyography in *Physical Medicine and Rehabilitation Clinics of North America*, GH Kraft, JJ Wertsch (eds.). Philadelphia, WB Saunders, 1998; pp 897–906.

Wagner AL, Buchthal F: Motor and sensory conduction in infancy and childhood: Reappraisal. *Dev Med Child Neurol* 14:189–216, 1972.

INDEX

A

Abdominal muscle strengthening, 61–62
Abductor digiti minimi (ulnar nerve), F waves of, 199–200
Abductor pollicis brevis (median nerve), F waves of, 198, 199*f*
Accommodation, 23
Acrocyanosis, in tetraplegia, 102
Action potential
  amplitude of, 135
  waveform of, 135–136
Alternating current (AC), 17
Amplitude, 1
  of action potential, 135
  current, in muscle strengthening, 30–31
  of electrotherapy, 22–23
  of H-reflex, 178
  peak, 23
  peak-to-peak, 20*f*, 23
Ankle, electrical stimulation of
  for edema from sprain, 92
  for hemiplegia in cerebral palsy, 277–278
Anode, 15
Anterior cruciate ligament (ACL) reconstruction, muscle strengthening after, 37–38, 41–42
  with arthroscopic surgery, 45–46
  with immobilized leg, 35–36
  of quadriceps and hamstring, 43–44
Antidromic, 131
Arm. *See also* Upper extremities
  electrical stimulation of
    after stroke, 262–263
    in C4-C5 tetraplegic, 234–235
    in C4 tetraplegic, voice-activated, 236
  motor points on, 10*f*, 11*f*
  muscle strengthening in, after Colle's fracture, 59–60

Arndt-Schultz law, 68
Artifact, stimulus, 134
Atrophy, prevention/retardation of, 58

B

Back, motor points on, 12*f*
Beat duration, 22
Biofeedback EMG, in stroke patients, 255
Biphasic current, 17
  train of, 21*f*
Biphasic waveform, 17–18, 19*f*
  asymmetrical, 18–19, 20*f*
  symmetrical, 17–18, 19*f*
Blink reflex, 203–206, 204*f*, 205*f*
  electrotherapy for, 204–205, 204*f*
    clinical applications of, 206
    electrode placement in, 204, 204*f*
    EMG set-up in, 204
    patient position in, 204
    technical comments on, 206
  normal values of, 205–206, 205*f*
Bone grafts, 70
Bone healing, with delayed union, 67–85. *See also* Fracture(s)
  Arndt-Schultz law and, 68
  capacitative coupled electrical stimulation for, 70
  in failed long bone fractures, 85
  in lower extremity stress fractures, in athletes, 82
  in recalcitrant nonunions, 83–84
  cyclic loading in, 67
  pulsed electromagnetic fields for, 68–71, 68*f*, 69*f*
  with bone grafts, 70
  with hip prostheses, loosened cemented, 80–81
  in knee, degenerative arthrosis of, after valgus tibial osteotomy, 72
  in metatarsal nonunion, proximal fifth, 73–74
  in pseudoarthrosis, chronic childhood, 78–79

Bone healing, with delayed union,
    pulsed electromagnetic fields
    for (*continued*)
        in tibial diaphyseal delayed
        union/nonunion, with
        non–weight-bearing cast,
        74–77
    Wolff's law and, 67
Burn wounds, chronic, 121
Bursitis, acute edema from, 95
Burst, 17*f,* 20*f,* 21
Burst duration, 22

C
C4-C5 tetraplegic, electrotherapy of,
    forearm and hand in,
    234–235
C7 injury, incomplete, electrotherapy
    of, gait in, 247–249
C4 tetraplegic, voice-activated electro-
    therapy of, arm and hand in,
    236
Capacitative coupled electrical stimula-
    tion, 70
    for long bone fractures, failed, 85
    for lower extremity stress fractures,
        in athletes, 82
    for recalcitrant nonunions, 83–84
Carbon rubber electrodes, 7
Cathode, 15
Cerebral palsy, electrotherapy for, 275
    with diplegia, 285–286
        during gait, 287–288
    with hemiplegia, 283–284, 285–286
        of ankle, 277–278
        during gait, 287–288
        of wrist, 279–280
            with dorsal wrist splint, 281–283
Cerebrovascular accident (CVA). *See*
    Stroke
Cervical kinesiologic H-reflex, 194–195
Cervical radiculopathy, 190
    bilateral, 190, 191*f*
Chondromalacia, muscle strengthening
    with, 51–52
Circulation problems, electrotherapy
    for, 89–103
    with acrocyanosis in tetraplegia, 102

    with diabetic polyneuropathy, 101
    with edema
        acute, 89
            from hematoma, bursitis, or
            hemarthroses, 95
        chronic, 90
            from venous insufficiency or
            lymphatic obstruction, 96
        distal limb, 97–98
        motor level
            in agonist and antagonist mus-
            cles, 94
        postacute, 93
        sensory level, 91
            of sprained ankle, 92
    with Raynaud's disease, 101
        sensory level, 103
    with spinal cord injury, in deep vein
        thrombosis prevention,
        99–100
Clonus, 215
Closed loop control configuration, 232
Conduction time, 136
Conduction velocity, 136–137
Contraindications, to electrotherapy, 1,
    2*t*–4*t*
Current
    alternating, 17
    biphasic, 17
        train of, 21*f*
    galvanic, 17
    high voltage pulsed, 17, 18*f,* 22, 26
        (*See also* High voltage pulsed
        current)
    interferential, 31–32
    low intensity direct, 23, 106
    low voltage direct
        for chronic skin ulcers, 122–123
        for ischemic skin ulcers, 124–127
    micro- (*See* Microcurrent)
    mode of, 21
    monophasic pulsed, 17, 17*f* (*See also*
        specific indications, e.g.,
        Wound healing)
    for muscle strengthening, 30–31
Current density, 7–8
Current of injury, 68, 105

Cycles per second (hertz, Hz), 17, 19
Cyclic loading, 67
Cycling, in spinal cord–injured patients
    aerobic, 230
    electrically induced, 230–231

D

Decline time, 26
Deep vein thrombosis prevention, in
    spinal cord–injured patients,
    99–100
Delayed union, 67
Diabetic polyneuropathy, 101
Diplegia, cerebral palsy, electrotherapy
    for, 285–286
    during gait, 288–289
Distal latency, 131, 132*f*, 134–135
Duchenne's muscular dystrophy, elec-
    trotherapy for, 273, 292
    functional gait in, 291
    parameters in, 274
Duration, 22
Duty cycle, 24–25, 255. *See also* Off-
    time; On-time; Ramp time
    in muscle stimulation, 29–30
    in muscle strengthening, 29–30
    post stroke, 254–255

E

Edema, electrotherapy for
    acute, 89
        from hematoma, bursitis, or
        hemarthroses, 95
    chronic, 90
        from venous insufficiency or lym-
        phatic obstruction, 96
    distal limb, garment electrode,
        97–98
    motor level
        in agonist and antagonist muscles,
        94
    postacute, 93
    sensory level, 91
        in sprained ankle, 92
Electrode
    placement of, 8
    selection of, 7–8
Electrode garments, 230
    for distal limb edema, 97–98

for spinal cord–injured patients, 230
    in standing and stepping, 239–241
Electromagnetic electrotherapy, after
    ACL reconstruction, 45–46
Electromyography (EMG), biofeed-
    back, in stroke patients, 255
Electrotherapy. *See also* specific appli-
    cations, e.g., Stroke
    amplitude of, 22–23
    contraindications and precautions
        for, 1, 2*t*–4*t*
    documentation of, 15
    duration of, 19*f,* 22
    duty cycle in, 24–25
    equipment for, 6–9
        electrode placement in, 8
        electrode selection for, 7–8
        inspection of, 6–7
        trigger/motor point location and,
        8–9
    examination for, 4
    frequency in, 1*f,* 19, 21–22
    history in, 4–6
    interval of, 22
    metric conversions in, 26–27
    on-off times in, 23–24, 24*f*
    on-time and off-time in, 24*f,* 25
    parameters in, 16
    patient procedures in, 9, 15
    phase in, 16–19, 17*f*–20*f* (*See also*
        Phase)
    polarity of, 15–16
    ramp time *vs.* on/off-time in, 25–26
    ramp-up and ramp-down time in,
        24*f,* 25
    terminology in, 1
    uses of, 1, 2*t*
Equipment, electrotherapy, 6–9
    electrode placement in, 8
    electrodes, selection for, 7–8
    inspection of, 6–7
    trigger/motor point location in, 8–9
Extensor digitorum brevis (peroneal
    nerve), F waves of, 200–202,
    201*f*
Extensor digitorum muscles, elec-
    trotherapy of, with cerebral
    palsy, 284–285

Extensor spasticity, 215
Extremities. *See* specific extremities,
    e.g., Forearm, Upper
    extremities

F
F waves, 175, 196–206
    in blink reflex, 203–206, 204*f*, 205*f*
    clinical applications of, 197–198
    of lower extremities, 200–203
        extensor digitorum brevis (per-
            oneal nerve), 200–202, 201*f*
        flexor hallucis brevis (tibial nerve),
            202–203, 203*f*
    origin of, 196–197
    pathway of, 197, 197*f*
    of upper extremities, 198–200
        abductor digiti minimi (ulnar
            nerve), 199–200
        abductor pollicis brevis (median
            nerve), 198, 199*f*
Fall time, 26
Faradic waveform, 19
Fatigue, during muscle strengthening,
    30
Favored posture (FP), 194
Femoral nerve conduction study,
    170–172, 170*f*, 171*f*
Flexor carpi radialis H-reflex, 186–189,
    187*f*, 188*f*
    clinical applications of, 189
    clinical perspectives on, 189
    electrical stimulation in, 187–188,
        188*f*
    EMG set-up for, 187
    history taking on, 186
    latency of, 186
    normal values of, 188
    patient position in, 187, 187*f*
    procedure for, 186–187
    recording electrode placement in,
        187, 188*f*
    technical comments on, 189
Flexor hallucis brevis (tibial nerve),
    F waves of, 202–203, 203*f*
Flexor spasticity, 215
Forearm, electrical stimulation of. *See
    also* Upper extremities
    after Colle's fracture, 59–60

after stroke, 262–263
    in C4-C5 tetraplegic, 234–235
Fracture(s)
    capacitative coupled electrical stimu-
        lation for
        long bone, failed, 85
        lower extremity stress, in athletes,
            82
    Colle's, electrical stimulation after,
        59–60
    delayed union of, 67
    healing of, 67–85 (*See also* Bone
        healing)
    negative electric currents at, 68
    nonunion of, 67
Frequency, 1, 1*f*, 19, 21–22

G
Gain, 133
Gait training, electrical stimulation in
    for C7 injury, incomplete, 247–249
    for cerebral palsy
        with diplegia, 287–288
        with hemiplegia, 287–288
    for Duchenne's muscular dystrophy,
        291
    for spinal cord–injured patients,
        243–245
    for stroke patients, heel switch acti-
        vated, 260–261
Galvanic current, 17
Garment electrode stimulation, 230
    for distal limb edema, 97–98
    for spinal cord–injured patients, 230
    in standing and stepping, 239–241

H
H-maximum, 179
H-reflexes, 175, 176–196
    amplitude of, 178
    intensity of, 178–179
    kinesiologic
        cervical, 194–195
        lumbosacral, 195–196
        for optimal spinal posture,
            193–194
        for radiculopathy treatment,
            189–193, 191*f*, 192*f* (*See also
            under* Radiculopathy)

latency of, 177, 177f, 178f
  of lower extremities, 179–186
    soleus, 179–183, 180f, 181f (See
      also Soleus H-reflex)
    vastus medialis, 183–186, 184f
      (See also Vastus medialis
      H-reflex)
  pathway for, 176, 176f
  postural modifications on, 189–190
  recording of, 177
  of upper extremities, flexor carpi
    radialis, 186–189, 187f, 188f
    (See also Flexor carpi radialis
    H-reflex)
  use of, 176
H-threshold, 178
H wave, 175, 176–196. See also
  H-reflexes
Hand, electrical stimulation of
  after stroke, 262–263
  antagonist muscle in, 225
  in C4-C5 tetraplegic, 234–235
  in C4 tetraplegic, voice-activated,
    236
Hand muscles, spastic, after stroke, 224
Head trauma, electrical stimulation
  after
  multichannel, 256
  for range of motion, 257–259
Helmholtz configuration, 69
Hemarthroses, acute edema from, 95
Hematoma, acute edema from, 95
Hemiparetic, antagonistic sensory
  stimulation in, 223
Hemiplegia, electrotherapy for. See
  also Stroke
  with cerebral palsy, 283–284,
    285–286
  of ankle, 277–278
  during gait, 287–288
  of wrist, 279–280
    with dorsal wrist splint,
      281–283
  heel switch activated, in gait training,
    260–261
  multichannel, 256
Hertz (Hz), 17, 19

High voltage pulsed current, 17, 18f,
  22, 26
  for chronic stage III ulcers, lower
    extremity, 120
  for pressure ulcers, in spinal
    cord–injured patients,
    118–119
Hip prostheses, loosened cemented,
  pulsed electromagnetic stimulation for, 80–81
Hoffman response, 175, 176–196. See
  also H-reflexes

I
Immobilized limb, postsurgical, muscle
  strengthening for, 50
  in ACL reconstruction, 35–36
  in quadriceps, 39–40
Intensity, 1, 22
  of H-reflexes, 178–179
Interburst interval, 21, 22
Interferential (interference) current,
  31–32
Interosseous (radial) nerve, motor
  nerve conduction of,
  156–158, 157f
Interphase interval, 22
Interpulse interval, 22
Interval, 22
Intrapulse interval, 22
Isometric exercise, with electrical stim-
  ulation, 30

K
Kinesiologic H-reflexes
  for optimal spinal posture, 193–194
  for radiculopathy treatment,
    189–193, 191f, 192f
Knee arthroplasty, muscle strengthening after
  to prevent extensor lag, 53–54
  to prevent muscle atrophy, 55
Knee degenerative arthrosis, valgus tibial osteotomy for, pulsed
  electromagnetic stimulation
  after, 72
Knee ligament surgery, muscle
  strengthening after, 41–42

L

L4 radiculopathy, 190
Late waves, 175–206
    blink reflex, 203–206, 204*f*, 205*f* (*See
        also* Blink reflex)
    F waves, 175, 196–206 (*See also*
        F waves)
    H-reflexes, 175, 176–196 (*See also*
        H-reflexes)
    M-response, 175
    origin of, 175
Latency
    to deflection, 131, 132*f*, 134–135
    distal, 131, 132*f*, 134–135
    of H-reflex, 177, 177*f*, 178*f*
    flexor carpi radialis, 186
    proximal, 136
Lateral plantar nerve conduction,
        motor, 166–168, 167*f*
Leg. *See also* Lower extremities
    motor points on
        back, 14*f*
        front, 13*f*
    peroneal nerve of, electric stimula-
        tion of, in cast, 275
Loading, cyclic, 67
Long bone fractures, failed, capacita-
        tive coupled electrical stimu-
        lation for, 85
Low intensity direct current (LIDC),
        23, 106
Low intensity stimulation (LIS), 23,
        106
Low voltage direct current
    for chronic skin ulcers, 122–123
    for ischemic skin ulcers, 124–127
Low voltage electrical stimulation, for
        chronic burn wounds, 121
Lower extremities
    F waves of, 200–203
        extensor digitorum brevis (per-
            oneal nerve), 200–202, 201*f*
        flexor hallucis brevis (tibial nerve),
            202–203, 203*f*
    H-reflexes of, 179–186
        soleus, 179–183, 180*f*, 181*f*
        vastus medialis, 183–186, 184*f*

    stress fractures of, in athletes, elec-
        trical stimulation for, 82
Lumbosacral kinesiologic H-reflex,
        195–196
Lymphatic obstruction, chronic edema
        from, 96

M

M-response, 175, 178
M wave, 175, 178
Maximum voluntary isometric contrac-
        tions (%MVIC), 31
Medial plantar nerve conduction,
        motor, 164*f*, 165*f*, 167*f*,
        168–170
Median nerve
    anatomy of, 139
    F waves of, 198, 199*f*
    injury sites in, 139
Median nerve conduction study
    motor, 140–142, 140*f*, 141*f*
    sensory, 140*f*, 142–145, 144*f*
        antidromic, 140*f*, 145–147, 146*f*
Meniscectomy, open, muscle strength-
        ening after, 48–49
Metatarsal nonunion, pulsed electro-
        magnetic stimulation for,
        73–74
Metric conversions, 26–27
Microcurrent, 23, 106
Monophasic pulsed current, 17, 17*f*,
        110, 111–112
    for wound healing, 110, 111–112
        chronic stage III, 116–117
        chronic stage III or IV, 113,
            114–115
Monophasic waveform, 16–17, 17*f*
Monopolar recording, 133
Motor level electrical stimulation
    for acrocyanosis in tetraplegia, 102
    for edema control
        in agonist and antagonist muscle, 94
        postacute, 93
    to increase vasodilation, in Ray-
        naud's disease or diabetic
        polyneuropathy, 101
    to prevent deep vein thrombosis,
        with spinal cord injury,
        99–100

Motor nerve conduction
  in children, 273
  of posterior interosseous (radial)
      nerve, 156–158, 157*f*
Motor points, 8–9, 10*f*–14*f*
  arm
    back, 11*f*
    front, 10*f*
  leg
    back, 14*f*
    front, 13*f*
  torso and back, 12*f*
Muscle, denervated, 209–210
  electrical stimulation of, 209–212
    contraindications for, 210
    current parameters in, 211
    electrode parameters in, 211–212
    optimal conditions for, 210–211
Muscle atrophy, prevention or retarda-
    tion of, 58
Muscle position, in muscle strengthen-
    ing electrotherapy, 31
Muscle strengthening, 29–64
  abdominal, 61–62
  after anterior cruciate ligament
      reconstruction, 41–42
    arthroscopic, 45–46
    with immobilized leg, 35–36
    in quadriceps and hamstring,
        43–44
  after anterior cruciate ligament
      surgery, 37–38
  after knee arthroplasty
    to prevent extensor lag, 53–54
    to prevent muscle atrophy, 55
  after knee ligament surgery, 41–42
  after meniscectomy, open, 48–49
  for atrophy prevention/retardation, 58
  with chondromalacia, 51–52
  current amplitude in, 30–31
  duty cycle in, 29–30
  electromagnetic, after arthroscopic
      ACL reconstruction, 45–46
  fatigue in, 30
  forearm, with Colle's fracture, 59–60
  of immobilized limb, postsurgical, 50
  interferential current in, 31–32
    isometric exercise in, 30
    muscle position in, 31
    %MVIC in, 30–31
    with patella subluxation or disloca-
        tion, 51–52
    protocols for, 29
    pulsed electromagnetic field, 47
    quadriceps
      with inability to perform maxi-
          mum voluntary isometric
          contractions, 56–57
      during postop immobilization,
          39–40
    quadriceps femoris, normal, 33–34
    torque/time index in, 31
    triceps surae, 63–64
Muscle tone, abnormal
  after cerebral vascular accident, 216
  after spinal cord injury, 215–216
  electrical stimulation of, 215–227
    after spinal cord injury
      incomplete, with isometric
          exercise, 220–221
      reciprocal, of spastic and antag-
          onistic muscles, 226–227
    to reduce spasticity, 219
    amplitude in, 216
    of antagonist muscle, 222
      after CVA, 224
      after CVA: hand muscles, 225
    in hemiparetic, 223
    parameters and settings in,
        217–218
Muscle twitch, 21
%MVIC, 30–31
Myelination, peripheral nerve, 273

N
Nerve conduction velocity, 131–174
  accuracy of, 138–139
  calculation of, 132
  electrode placement in, 137
  femoral nerve, 170–172, 170*f*, 171*f*
  measurement of, 131–132, 133*f*
    filter setting in, 134
    sensitivity/gain in, 133
    sweep speed in, 134

Nerve conduction velocity (*continued*)
    median nerve, 139
        motor, 140–142, 140*f*, 141*f*
        sensory, 140*f*, 142–145, 144*f*
        sensory antidromic, 140*f*,
            145–147, 146*f*
    motor nerve, 131, 132*f*
    posterior interosseous (radial)
        nerve, 156–158, 157*f*
    orthodromic action potentials in, 131
    parameters of studies of, 134–137
        action potential amplitude, 135
        action potential waveform,
            135–136
        conduction time, 136
        conduction velocity, 136–137
        distal latency, 132*f*, 134–135
        proximal latency, 136
        stimulus artifact, 134
    peroneal nerve, motor, 160–163,
        161*f*, 162*f*
    plantar nerve, motor
        lateral, 166–168, 167*f*
        medial, 164*f*, 165*f*, 167*f*, 168–170
    radial nerve, sensory, 157*f*, 159–160,
        159*f*
    Roth technique for
        in median (sensory) orthodromic
            nerve, 143, 144*f*
        in ulnar (sensory) orthodromic
            nerve, 151, 153*f*
    sural nerve, sensory, 161*f*, 172–174,
        173*f*
    tibial nerve, motor, 163–166, 164*f*, 165*f*
    ulnar nerve, 148–150, 148*f*, 149*f*
        anatomic considerations in,
            147–148
        sensory antidromic, 140*f*, 154–155,
            155*f*
        sensory orthodromic, 140*f*, 150–154,
            152*f*, 153*f*
Nonunion, 67
    recalcitrant, electrical stimulation
        for, 83–84

O
Off-time, 24, 24*f*, 25
    vs. ramp time, 25–26

On/off times, 23–24, 24*f*
On-time, 23–24, 24*f*, 25
    vs. ramp time, 25–26
Open loop control configuration,
    231–232
Optimal spinal posture (OSP), deter-
    mination of, 191, 193–194
Orthodromic, 131

P
Parameters, 16
Patella subluxation/dislocation, muscle
    strengthening for, 51–52
Peak amplitude, 23
Peak-to-peak amplitude, 20*f*, 23
Pediatric electrotherapy, 273–300
    for cerebral palsy, 275
        with diplegia, 286–287
            during gait, 288–289
        with hemiplegia, 284–285,
            286–287
            of ankle, 277–278
                during gait, 288–289
            of wrist, 279–280
            of wrist, with dorsal wrist splint,
                281–283
    for Duchenne's muscular dystrophy,
        273, 274, 293
    functional gait in, 292
    guidelines for, 275–276
    indications for, 273
    injury etiology and, 274
    motor nerve conduction velocities
        and, 273
    nerve myelination and, 273
    for scoliosis
        idiopathic, 299
        lateral, 295
        thoracic, 297–298
        at night, with daytime bracing, 296
    for spina bifida, 289–290
Peroneal nerve
    electric stimulation of, 256
        heel switch activated, 260–261
        in pediatric leg cast, 275
    F waves of, 200–202, 201*f*
    motor conduction study of, 160–163,
        161*f*, 162*f*
    in children, 273

Phase, 16–19, 17f–20f
    in biphasic waveform, 17–18, 19f
        asymmetrical, 18–19, 20f
        symmetrical, 17–18, 19f
    in high voltage pulsed current, 17,
        18f, 22, 26
    in monophasic pulsed current, 17, 17f
    in monophasic waveform, 16–17, 17f
Phase duration, 19f, 22
Plantar nerve conduction study, motor
    lateral, 166–168, 167f
    medial, 164f, 165f, 167f, 168–170
Polarity, 15–16
Posterior interosseous (radial) nerve,
    motor nerve conduction of,
    156–158, 157f
Precautions, in electrotherapy, 1, 2t–4t
Premature birth, cerebral palsy from,
    293–294
Pressure ulcers, in spinal cord–injured
    patients, 118–119
Proximal latency, 136
Pseudoarthrosis, chronic childhood,
    78–79
Pulse, 22
Pulsed electromagnetic fields
    (PEMFs), 47, 68–71, 68f, 69f
    bone grafts with, 70
    for hip prostheses, loosened
        cemented, 80–81
    for knee, degenerative arthrosis of,
        after valgus tibial osteotomy,
        72
    for metatarsal nonunion, proximal
        fifth, 73–74
    for pseudoarthrosis, chronic child-
        hood, 78–79
    for tibial diaphyseal delayed union/
        nonunion, with non–weight-
        bearing cast, 74–77
Pulses per second (pps), 17

Q
Quadriceps, muscle strengthening of
    with inability to perform maximum
        voluntary isometric contrac-
        tions, 56–57
    during postop immobilization, 39–40

Quadriceps femoris, muscle strength-
    ening of, 33–34

R
Radial nerve conduction study, sensory,
    157f, 159–160, 159f
Radiculopathy
    H-reflex latency in, 177
    kinesiologic H-reflexes for, 189–193,
        191f, 192f
        in cervical radiculopathy, 190
            bilateral, 190, 191f
        in favored vs. unfavored postures,
            193
        in L4 radiculopathy, 190
        in lying position, 190, 192f
        in optimal spinal posture, 191,
            193–194
        in remyelination monitoring, 193
        in sitting or standing position, 190,
            192f
    postural modifications and, 189–190
Ramp-down time, 24f, 25
Ramp time, 30
    vs. on/off-time, 25–26
Ramp-up time, 24f, 25
Rate, 19
Raynaud's disease, 101
Reflex sympathetic dystrophy (RSD;
    shoulder-hand syndrome),
    after stroke, 253–254
Rolling walker/stimulation systems, 231
    closed loop control configuration of,
        232
    open loop control configuration of,
        231–232
Roth technique
    for median (sensory) orthodromic
        nerve conduction, 143, 144f
    for ulnar (sensory) orthodromic
        nerve conduction, 151, 153f
Russian stimulation, 22, 25, 29

S
Scoliosis, electrotherapy for
    with idiopathic disease, 299
    lateral, 295
        thoracic, 297–298
    at night, with daytime bracing, 296

Self-adhesive disposable electrodes, 7
Sensitivity/gain, 133
Sensory level electrical stimulation,
    103. *See also* specific sites
    and indications, e.g., Ulnar
    nerve, Edema
Shoulder-hand syndrome (Reflex Sym-
    pathetic Dystrophy), after
    stroke, 253–254
Shoulder subluxation, after stroke, 253
  electrical stimulation to prevent,
    264–265
  with flaccid shoulder, 266–267
  electrical stimulation to treat, 268–269
Skin ulcers
  chronic, 122–123
    stage III, lower extremity, 120
    stage III or IV, 113, 114–115
    ischemic, 124–127
    pressure, in spinal cord–injured
      patients, 118–119
Soleus H-reflex, 179–183, 180*f*, 181*f*
  clinical application of, 182
  clinical perspectives on, 182–183
  electrical parameters for, 181, 181*f*
  EMG setup for, 180
  kinesiologic, 195–196
  normal values of, 181
  patient position for, 180, 180*f*
  procedure for, 179–180
  recording electrode placement for,
    181, 181*f*
  technical comments on, 182
Spasticity, 215
  extensor, 215
  flexor, 215
  reduction of, with spinal cord injury,
    219
  treatment of, 216
Spina bifida, pediatric electrotherapy
  for, 289–290
Spinal cord–injured patients
  abnormal muscle tone in, 215–216
  electrical stimulation of, 229–249
    for ambulation, 231
    with C7 injury, for gait, 247–249
    for cycling
      aerobic, 230
      electrically induced, 230–231

for deep vein thrombosis preven-
    tion, 99–100
  effects of, 229
  electrode garments for, 230
    in standing and stepping,
      239–241
    for gait swing, 243–245
    heel switch for, with incomplete
      injury, 232
    hybrid systems of, 232–233
    incomplete, with isometric exer-
      cise, 220–221
    muscle fatigue from, 229–230
    in paraplegic, for standing, 246
    patient evaluation for, 233
    for pressure ulcers, 118–119
    reciprocal, of spastic and antago-
      nistic muscles, 226–227
    rolling walker/stimulation systems
      for, 231
      closed loop control configura-
        tion of, 232
      open loop control configuration
        of, 231–232
    for spasticity, 219
    standing with, static, 231
    with T5-T6 spinal lesion, to
      induce standing, 237–238
    in tetraplegic, 232
    in tetraplegic, C4, of arm and
      hand, voice-activated, 236
    in tetraplegic, C4-C5, of forearm
      and hand, 234–235
    tibialis anterior, to increase fatigue
      resistance, 242
  muscle changes in, 229
  muscle tone in, 215–216
Spinal posture, optimal, 191, 193–194
Sponge electrodes, 7
Standing
  with radiculopathy, kinesiologic
    H-reflexes for, 190, 192*f*
  in spinal cord–injured patients
    electrical stimulation for, 231, 246
      with T5-T6 spinal lesion, 237–238
    electrode garments for, 239–241
Stepping, electrode garments for, with
    spinal cord injury, 239–241

Stimulus artifact, 134
Stress fractures, lower extremity, electrical stimulation for, 82
Stroke (cerebrovascular accident), 216
  electrical stimulation after, 253–269
    of antagonistic muscle, 224
    duty cycle in, 254–255
    of forearm and hand, 262–263
    in gait training, heel switch activated, 260–261
    multichannel, 256
    plus EMG biofeedback, 255
    for range of motion, 257–259
    remote switches for, 255–256, 260–261
    for shoulder subluxation prevention, 264–265
      for flaccid shoulder, 266–267
      for shoulder subluxation treatment, 268–269
    of spastic hand muscles, 224
  range-of-motion exercises after, 254
  reflex sympathetic dystrophy after, 253–254
    electrotherapy prevention of, 254
  shoulder subluxation after, 253
    electrotherapy prevention of, 254
Sural nerve conduction study, sensory, 161f, 172–174, 173f
Sweep speed, 134

T

T5-T6 spinal lesion, electrotherapy for, to induce standing, 237–238
Tetany, 21
Tetraplegic patients
  acrocyanosis in, 102
  electrical stimulation of, 232
Tibial diaphyseal delayed union/nonunion, with non–weight-bearing cast, pulsed electromagnetic stimulation for, 74–77
Tibial nerve, F waves of, 202–203, 203f
Tibial nerve conduction
  in children, 273
  motor, 163–166, 164f, 165f
Tibialis anterior, electrotherapy of
  with cerebral palsy, 283–284

with Duchenne's muscular dystrophy, 291
Torque/time index, 31
Torso, motor points on, 12f
Train, 21, 21f
Triceps surae, strengthening of, 63–64
Trigger points, 8–9
Twitch, muscle, 21

U

Ulcers. See specific types, e.g., Skin ulcers
Ulnar nerve, F waves of, 199–200
Ulnar nerve conduction study, 148–150, 148f, 149f
  anatomic considerations in, 147–148
  sensory antidromic, 140f, 154–155, 155f
  sensory orthodromic, 140f, 150–154, 152f, 153f
Unfavored posture (UP), 194
Unwanted spinal posture (USP), 194
Upper extremities
  F waves of, 198–200
    abductor digiti minimi (ulnar nerve), 199–200
    abductor pollicis brevis (median nerve), 198, 199f
  H-reflexes of, 186–189, 187f, 188f

V

Vastus medialis H-reflex, 183–186, 184f
  clinical applications of, 185
  clinical perspectives on, 186
  electrical stimulation for, 184–185, 184f
  electrode placement for, 184, 184f
  EMG set-up for, 184
  kinesiologic, 195–196
  normal values of, 185
  patient position for, 184
  protocol for, 183
  technical comments on, 185
Venous insufficiency, chronic edema from, 96

W

Waveform(s)
  biphasic, 17–18, 19f

Waveform(s) (*continued*)
    asymmetrical, 18–19, 20*f*
    symmetrical, 17–18, 19*f*
    monophasic, 16–17, 17*f*
Wolff's law, 67
Wound healing, 105–127
    current of injury in, 105
    disease control measures in, 107–108
    documentation of, 108–109
    electrode configuration for, 109
    high voltage pulsed current for
        with chronic stage III ulcers,
            lower extremity, 120
        with pressure ulcers, spinal cord
            injury, 118–119
    infection type in, 106–107
    low voltage direct current for
        with chronic skin ulcers, 122–123
    with ischemic skin ulcers, 124–127
    low voltage electrical stimulation for,
        with chronic burn wounds,
            121
    monophasic pulsed current for, 110,
        111–112
    with chronic stage III wounds,
        116–117
    with skin ulcer, chronic stage III
        or IV, 113, 114–115
    procedure for, 108
    protocol for, 106–107
    through wound dressing, 105–106
Wrist, electrical stimulation of, for
        hemiplegia in cerebral palsy,
        279–280
    with dorsal wrist splint, 281–283

ISBN 0-07-134317-2

90000

9 780071 343176